Chapter 1: Understanding Calories

1.1 What Are Calories, and Why Do They Matter?

Calories are often seen as the enemy when it comes to weight loss. We hear phrases like "calorie bombs" or "burning calories," and it's easy to develop a negative association. But at their core, calories are simply a unit of energy—just like how we measure distance in miles or kilometers. Calories provide the energy our bodies need to function, from breathing and thinking to physical activities like walking or exercising. Every time you eat food, you're providing your body with energy in the form of calories.

Your body needs a certain amount of energy every day just to keep functioning. This is known as your **Basal Metabolic Rate (BMR)**—the number of calories required for basic bodily functions like breathing, maintaining body temperature, and keeping your heart beating. Beyond this, any physical activity you do—from walking to dancing—burns additional calories. Understanding how many calories your body needs is the key to weight loss.

1.2 Calories In, Calories Out (CICO): The Simple Science Behind Weight Loss

The fundamental concept of weight loss boils down to something called **Calories In, Calories Out (CICO)**. If you consistently take in more calories than your body needs, those extra calories get stored as fat. If you consume fewer calories than you need, your body turns to stored fat to make up the difference, which is how weight loss occurs. In simple terms:

- **Calories In > Calories Out**: Weight gain.
- **Calories In < Calories Out**: Weight loss.

- **Calories In = Calories Out**: Weight maintenance.

For many people, this simple principle can be life-changing. By creating a calorie deficit—eating fewer calories than your body burns—you can lose weight without having to give up your favorite foods.

1.3 Your Personal Calorie Needs

Everyone's body is different, and so are their calorie needs. Factors like age, gender, height, weight, and activity level all influence how many calories you need. To determine how many calories you should be eating, you need to understand two main components: your **Basal Metabolic Rate (BMR)** and your **Total Daily Energy Expenditure (TDEE)**.

- **Basal Metabolic Rate (BMR)**: This is the number of calories your body burns at rest, just to keep your organs functioning. You can calculate an estimate of your BMR using various online calculators or formulas like the **Mifflin-St Jeor Equation**. For example, a moderately active 30-year-old woman who weighs 150 pounds and is 5'5" tall might have a BMR of around 1,400 calories.

- **Total Daily Energy Expenditure (TDEE)**: Your TDEE takes your BMR and adds the calories burned through daily activities and exercise. It's a more accurate measure of how many calories you actually need in a day. Using our example, if the same 30-year-old woman is moderately active, her TDEE might be around 2,000 calories. This means she needs 2,000 calories per day to maintain her current weight.

To lose weight, you'll want to create a calorie deficit—generally aiming for 500 calories fewer per day than your TDEE, which can lead to a weight loss of about 1 pound per week. This deficit can be achieved by eating fewer calories, burning more through exercise, or a combination of both.

1.4 Why Restriction Doesn't Work: The Case for Flexibility

Most people struggle with weight loss because they think they have to eliminate all their favorite foods. They try diets that make burgers, fried chicken, and even bread seem like forbidden pleasures. The problem with restrictive diets is that they're not sustainable. They leave you feeling deprived, which often leads to binge eating or giving up entirely.

The key to sustainable weight loss is **flexibility**. Instead of seeing foods as "good" or "bad," think of them in terms of calories and balance. Burgers and fried chicken are higher in calories, but that doesn't mean you can't eat them. You just have to learn how to fit them into your daily calorie budget. By understanding your calorie needs, you can make informed choices and build meals that work for you—without guilt or deprivation.

1.5 The Energy Balance Equation: Inputs and Outputs

To get a clearer picture of calories in your life, think of your body like a bank account. The calories you eat are your deposits, while the calories you burn are your withdrawals. Just as you might track your finances to save for a goal, you can track your calories to manage your weight. The balance of calories in versus calories out is what determines whether you'll lose, gain, or maintain your weight.

One thing to remember is that calorie needs can vary day by day based on your activity levels. On more active days, you might burn more calories, while on less active days, your needs might be lower. By maintaining awareness of your general needs and making adjustments as needed, you can ensure that you stay on track while still allowing for treats.

1.6 The Importance of Calorie Density

Another concept that can help you understand calories is **calorie density**. Some foods are calorie-dense, meaning they contain a lot of calories in a small amount. Examples include fried foods, baked goods, and sugary drinks. Other foods, like vegetables, fruits, and lean proteins, have fewer calories for a larger volume, making them less calorie-dense.

This doesn't mean you should avoid calorie-dense foods altogether. In fact, they can be very satisfying when you're craving something rich and flavorful. However, understanding which foods are calorie-dense can help you plan more balanced meals and make smarter choices throughout the day. For instance, if you know you're having a burger for dinner, you can balance your other meals to accommodate it—like having a big, nutrient-dense salad for lunch that fills you up without using too many of your daily calories.

1.7 Tracking Calories Without Stress

One of the most effective ways to understand and manage your calorie intake is through **tracking**. While it may sound tedious, modern technology has made tracking easier than ever. There are numerous apps available that allow you to simply scan a barcode or search for a food to log its calories. These apps can also provide you with information about macronutrients (proteins, fats, carbs) and help you understand your eating habits better.

Tracking your calories doesn't mean you have to be obsessive or overly restrictive. It's about awareness and understanding. You might be surprised at how certain foods add up or how small changes can have a big impact. For example, swapping a regular soda for a diet soda could save you 150 calories, which adds up over time. Tracking can help you identify these opportunities for change without making you feel like you're on a diet.

1.8 Finding Your Balance: A Real-Life Example

Imagine that you've calculated your TDEE to be 2,000 calories per day. To create a deficit and lose weight, you decide to aim for 1,500 calories per day. How do you fit in your favorite foods?

Let's say you're craving a burger. A typical fast-food burger might have around 500 calories. You can still have it! The key is to balance the rest of your day accordingly:

- **Breakfast**: Instead of a high-calorie breakfast, opt for something lighter, like a bowl of Greek yogurt with fruit (around 250 calories).

- **Lunch**: Have a nutrient-dense salad with lots of vegetables, some grilled chicken, and a light dressing (around 300 calories).

- **Dinner**: Enjoy your burger (500 calories) with a side of roasted vegetables instead of fries.

- **Snacks**: Have some fresh fruit or a handful of nuts throughout the day (200-250 calories).

By planning your meals this way, you still get to enjoy the burger without exceeding your daily calorie target. Over time, this balance becomes second nature, allowing you to incorporate the foods you love while staying on track with your goals.

1.9 Why This Approach Is Sustainable

The reason calorie counting works so well for many people is that it's not about giving up what you enjoy. It's about being mindful and making informed decisions. You get to have burgers, fried chicken, pizza, and all the things that make life delicious—just in moderation. This way, you don't feel deprived, and you're much more likely to stick to your plan in the long run.

Instead of seeing food as a battleground, you begin to see it as a source of joy and energy. You learn that it's not about avoiding calories; it's about managing them in a way that aligns with your goals. By understanding calories, you take control of your diet and your health, making it possible to lose weight without losing your love for food.

Chapter 2: The Tools You Need

2.1 Embracing Technology: The Calorie Tracking Revolution

In the past, managing calories and keeping track of your diet was a cumbersome task, often requiring tedious calculations and food diaries. But in today's world, technology has made the process not only more accessible but even enjoyable. In this chapter, we'll cover the essential tools that will help you stay on track, plan your meals, and make your weight-loss journey more manageable.

First and foremost, calorie tracking apps have become the go-to solution for anyone wanting to lose weight without drastic lifestyle changes. Apps like **MyFitnessPal**, **Lose It!**, and **Cronometer** allow you to log your meals and easily track calories and nutrients. These apps have vast food databases with nutritional information for almost any food you can imagine, making tracking as simple as typing in a name or scanning a barcode. These tools are indispensable for understanding how your daily habits affect your calorie intake and overall progress.

The key to using these apps successfully is consistency. Logging what you eat every day, even when it's not perfect, will give you an accurate picture of where you are and what adjustments might be needed. Remember, these tools are not there to judge you—they are there to empower you, to help you make better decisions without taking away the foods you love.

2.2 Measuring Success Beyond the Scale

Weight loss isn't just about the number on the scale. For many, focusing solely on the scale can be frustrating, especially when you hit those inevitable plateaus. One way to keep motivated and track your progress in a healthier way is to use multiple measures of success.

Consider using these tools:

- **Body Measurements**: Get a tape measure and take regular measurements of your waist, hips, chest, and other parts of your body. Sometimes, even when the scale doesn't move, you'll notice inches melting away. This is a great indicator that you're making progress, especially when strength training is involved.

- **Progress Photos**: Take photos of yourself every few weeks. Progress can often be more visible in photos than on the scale, giving you a sense of achievement that keeps you motivated.

- **Fitness Trackers**: Devices like **Fitbit**, **Apple Watch**, or **Garmin** can help you monitor your physical activity, steps, and calories burned throughout the day. While you don't need to over-focus on every single step, having an overview of your activity level can help you maintain a balance between energy in and energy out.

These tools are valuable in helping you shift the focus away from just weight and instead emphasize the bigger picture of health and well-being.

2.3 Kitchen Essentials: Keeping it Simple and Delicious

Part of succeeding in your weight loss journey is having a kitchen equipped with the right tools to make cooking easy and enjoyable. Here are some essential kitchen items that can help you create tasty, satisfying meals without much fuss:

- **Food Scale**: One of the most important tools in your kitchen should be a **food scale**. It helps you accurately measure portion sizes, which is essential for tracking calories. Many people underestimate the amount of food they eat, so having a scale will give you an accurate understanding of your portions.

- **Measuring Cups and Spoons**: While a food scale is the most precise, measuring cups and spoons are also helpful for items like liquids or when you're cooking larger quantities. They help you stick to proper portion sizes and prevent accidental overeating.

- **Non-Stick Cookware**: Cooking methods play a significant role in the number of calories a dish has. Using **non-stick pans** can significantly reduce the need for added fats like butter or oil. This way, you can save on unnecessary calories without compromising on flavor.

- **Air Fryer**: An **air fryer** can be a game-changer for those who love fried foods but want to cut down on calories. It allows you to cook crispy, "fried" foods with very little oil, providing the taste and texture you crave without the extra calories. Fried chicken, anyone?

- **Blender or Immersion Blender**: Making your own smoothies, dressings, or soups can be a great way to enjoy nutrient-dense foods that are lower in calories. A **blender** or **immersion blender** helps you whip up these delicious options in minutes.

By keeping these essentials handy, you'll be prepared to make nutritious and satisfying meals that fit your calorie budget, all while enjoying the foods you love.

2.4 Grocery Shopping Tips: Stocking Up for Success

Success starts with the foods you have at home. If your pantry is filled with calorie-dense, high-sugar snacks, then staying within your calorie budget can be a challenge. However, with some strategic shopping, you can still stock your kitchen with foods you love while making smart choices that help you stay on track.

- **Plan Ahead**: Planning your meals for the week can help you make a clear grocery list. By sticking to your list, you'll be less likely to make impulse purchases that may derail your progress. Plus, having a plan reduces stress around mealtimes.

- **Read Labels**: Understanding nutrition labels is key to making good choices. Check the calorie content per serving, and pay attention to the portion size listed. You'd be surprised how often serving sizes are much smaller than what we might usually eat. Look for options that align with your goals—foods that are high in protein or fiber are great for keeping you full.

- **Calorie-Friendly Staples**: Stock up on items that are versatile and can be used to create a variety of meals. These include:

  - **Lean Proteins**: Chicken breast, turkey, fish, tofu, eggs, and low-fat dairy are great protein options that are satisfying and lower in calories.

  - **Vegetables and Fruits**: Low in calories but high in nutrients and fiber, vegetables and fruits help fill you up without blowing your calorie budget.

  - **Whole Grains**: Foods like oats, quinoa, brown rice, and whole-wheat bread can be filling and provide lasting energy.

  - **Low-Calorie Condiments**: Sugar-free ketchup, mustard, hot sauce, and vinegar-based dressings can add a lot of flavor without adding many calories.

- **Be Flexible**: Remember, there's room for indulgence. Buy that box of cookies if it fits your calorie budget—just be mindful of the portions and make them part of a balanced diet. This book isn't about restriction; it's about making your favorite foods fit your goals.

2.5 Meal Prep for Real Life: Keeping It Simple and Tasty

Meal prepping often sounds intimidating, but it doesn't have to mean spending hours in the kitchen. Meal prep is simply a way to make it easier to stick to your calorie goals throughout the week by having nutritious and satisfying options readily available.

- **Batch Cooking**: Cook larger portions of proteins like grilled chicken or roasted vegetables, then use them in multiple dishes throughout the week. One batch of chicken could be used in salads, sandwiches, wraps, or even as part of a stir-fry.

- **Mix and Match**: Think of meal prepping like creating building blocks. Prepare different components—like cooked grains, chopped vegetables, and proteins—that you can mix and match throughout the week to create different meals. This approach keeps things from getting boring while still being efficient.

- **Portion Control**: One of the benefits of meal prepping is that you can portion out your meals ahead of time. This way, you're not tempted to overeat when you're hungry. By having your meals ready in the right portions, sticking to your calorie goals becomes much easier.

- **Snack Prep**: Pre-packaged snacks can often be high in calories and low in nutrients. Preparing your own snacks, like sliced vegetables with hummus or a small portion of nuts, ensures that you have satisfying options when hunger strikes.

Meal prepping doesn't have to be complicated or time-consuming. It's about finding ways to make it easier to eat well and stay on track with your calorie goals, especially when life gets busy.

2.6 Navigating Social Situations and Eating Out

One of the biggest challenges for people trying to lose weight is eating out or attending social events. It can be difficult to gauge calorie content when you're not in control of the cooking, but there are some great strategies to help you navigate these situations.

- **Look Up Menus in Advance**: Many restaurants provide nutritional information online. Look up the menu ahead of time, and decide what fits your calorie goals before you go. This way, you won't feel overwhelmed by the options when you're there.

- **Make Adjustments**: Don't be afraid to ask for modifications to your meal. Requesting dressings or sauces on the side, asking for grilled instead of fried, or swapping out a side for a salad are all small changes that can make a big difference in calorie count.

- **Balance Your Day**: If you know you'll be eating out for dinner, plan your other meals accordingly. Opt for lower-calorie, nutrient-dense foods during the day to give yourself more room for indulgence at dinner.

- **Listen to Your Hunger Cues**: Eating out often means larger portion sizes, and we can feel obligated to clean our plates. Practice mindful eating by listening to your hunger and fullness cues. Eat slowly, enjoy your food, and stop when you're satisfied—even if that means taking leftovers home.

2.7 Mindset Tools: Staying Motivated and Consistent

Weight loss is as much a mental challenge as it is a physical one. The tools you need for success aren't just about tracking calories or cooking at home—they're also about building a mindset that will keep you consistent.

- **Progress Not Perfection**: Understand that nobody is perfect. You will have days where you eat more than you intended or when your meal doesn't go as planned. The key is to get back on track without guilt or self-punishment. Progress is made by staying consistent over the long term, not by being perfect every day.

- **Set Realistic Goals**: Having clear, achievable goals helps keep you focused. These could be related to weight loss, like losing 1 pound a week, or behavior-based goals, like tracking your food every day or eating more vegetables. Setting goals that are realistic ensures you don't get discouraged.

- **Celebrate Small Wins**: Every step forward counts. Celebrate your progress, whether it's a weight milestone, a healthier food swap, or just staying on track during a tough day. Recognizing these small victories can keep you motivated to continue your journey.

- **Self-Compassion**: Weight loss can be challenging, and there will be setbacks. Practicing self-compassion means treating yourself with kindness, just as you would a friend who's struggling. It's okay to stumble; what matters is getting up and moving forward.

Chapter 3: Crafting a Balanced Plate: Enjoying Your Favorite Foods While Staying on Track

3.1 Why Balance Matters: Fueling Your Body for Success

When it comes to weight loss, many people make the mistake of only focusing on eating less without considering the quality of what they're eating. But focusing on balance is crucial for a few reasons:

- **Nutrient Needs**: Your body needs a variety of nutrients to function at its best. Carbohydrates, proteins, fats, vitamins, and minerals all have specific roles. A balanced plate ensures that you're getting the energy, nutrition, and satisfaction you need, making it easier to stick to your goals without feeling deprived or fatigued.

- **Satiety and Hunger Control**: Balanced meals help keep you full and satisfied longer, which reduces the temptation to overeat. Protein and fiber, in particular, are known for promoting satiety and managing hunger hormones. By learning to craft a balanced plate, you'll naturally find it easier to stay within your calorie budget without feeling constantly hungry or deprived.

- **Sustaining Energy Levels**: When your meals are balanced, you'll maintain consistent energy throughout the day. An unbalanced meal—like one filled only with refined carbs—can lead to spikes and crashes in energy, leaving you feeling tired and sluggish. With balance, you get a steady release of energy that keeps you feeling strong and motivated.

This chapter is all about making sure your body gets what it needs while still leaving room for the indulgences you love. Let's get started on crafting a balanced plate that helps you feel great and reach your weight loss goals.

3.2 The Components of a Balanced Plate

A balanced plate should contain a mix of **protein, healthy fats, carbohydrates**, and plenty of **fiber** (mostly from vegetables and fruits). Let's break down each component and understand its role in crafting meals that are not only nutritious but also satisfying.

- **Protein**: This is perhaps the most important component for anyone looking to lose weight. Protein is known for keeping you full, building and maintaining lean muscle mass, and aiding in recovery from physical activity. Aim to have a source of protein in every meal—this could be anything from chicken, fish, tofu, beans, eggs, to dairy products. Including protein at every meal will keep you feeling satisfied for longer, reducing the need to snack between meals.

- **Carbohydrates**: Carbohydrates are often unfairly demonized in diet culture, but they are an important source of energy. The key is to focus on complex carbohydrates that are rich in fiber and slow-digesting, such as whole grains, legumes, starchy vegetables, and fruits. These carbs provide lasting energy, help with digestion, and contribute to feeling full and satisfied.

- **Healthy Fats**: Healthy fats are crucial for hormone function, satiety, and the absorption of fat-soluble vitamins. Adding fats like avocado, olive oil, nuts, seeds, or fatty fish to your meal can make it more enjoyable and keep you full for longer. Fats are also calorie-dense, which means they need to be portioned out mindfully. However, they play a key role in keeping your meals flavorful and satisfying.

- **Fiber**: Fiber is your secret weapon when it comes to staying full and satisfied while losing weight. It aids digestion, slows down the release of sugar into your bloodstream, and keeps you feeling full. Vegetables and fruits are excellent sources of fiber, as well as being low in calories. The more non-starchy vegetables you include in your meals, the fuller you'll feel without consuming a large number of calories.

3.3 Building Your Plate: Practical Examples

Now that you understand the key components of a balanced plate, let's look at some practical examples. Crafting a balanced plate means including a mix of these components to provide a range of flavors and textures while keeping you within your calorie goal.

- **The Classic Burger Plate**: A burger doesn't have to be off-limits. Here's how you can craft a balanced meal that includes a burger:

  - **Protein**: Start with a lean beef patty (around 90% lean) or even a turkey burger for fewer calories. Protein will be the star of your plate.

  - **Carbohydrate**: Instead of a large bun, you can opt for a whole-wheat bun or even use lettuce wraps to reduce calories.

  - **Healthy Fats**: Add a slice of cheese or avocado. Be mindful of portions—just a small amount goes a long way in adding flavor.

  - **Fiber and Veggies**: Load up your burger with plenty of veggies—lettuce, tomato, onion, pickles, and mushrooms. On the side, have a big salad with a light vinaigrette or roasted veggies to fill you up without adding many calories.

- **The Fried Chicken Plate**: Yes, you can have fried chicken!

  - **Protein**: Choose a smaller portion of fried chicken. Alternatively, try making it at home in an **air fryer** for that crispy texture without the excess oil.

  - **Carbohydrate**: Pair it with a moderate serving of roasted potatoes or sweet potatoes. The key is to keep portions in check to fit within your calorie goals.

- o   **Healthy Fats**: The chicken will likely have some fat already, especially if it's fried, so you may not need to add extra.

  - o   **Fiber and Veggies**: Balance out the fried chicken with a large side of non-starchy vegetables, such as steamed broccoli or a crunchy coleslaw with a light yogurt-based dressing. This keeps your meal satisfying while ensuring you're still getting essential nutrients.

- **The Balanced Breakfast Plate**: Breakfast can be tough, especially with high-calorie options like sugary cereals or pastries. Here's a balanced take:

  - o   **Protein**: Greek yogurt or eggs.

  - o   **Carbohydrate**: A slice of whole-grain toast or a serving of oats. Add some berries for natural sweetness.

  - o   **Healthy Fats**: Top your toast with a small serving of nut butter or sprinkle some nuts on your yogurt.

  - o   **Fiber**: Make sure to include fruit or vegetables—berries in your oats or sautéed veggies with your eggs.

3.4 Indulgence Days and How to Fit in Your Favorites

Weight loss doesn't mean saying goodbye to your favorite high-calorie meals. Instead, it's about learning how to fit them into your weekly plan so you can indulge without falling off track.

- **Planned Indulgences**: Plan for a meal where you eat what you truly crave—a juicy burger, fried chicken, pizza, or even dessert. By planning for indulgences, you're less likely to feel deprived, which reduces the risk of binging. If you know Friday night is your burger night, you're more likely to stick to your balanced meals during the week because you have something to look forward to.

- **Adjusting Your Day**: When you know an indulgent meal is coming, adjust the rest of your day to accommodate it. For example, if you're planning on having fried chicken for dinner, you can keep breakfast and lunch lighter and more nutrient-dense. This doesn't mean starving yourself—it means filling up on low-calorie, high-volume foods like vegetables, fruits, and lean proteins earlier in the day to leave room for the indulgent meal later.

- **Portion Control**: You don't always have to eat an entire serving. Sometimes, sharing a portion or saving half for later can allow you to enjoy what you love without consuming too many calories at once. Enjoy the flavors, eat slowly, and savor every bite.

3.5 Healthy Cooking Techniques for Maximum Flavor

Cooking at home gives you more control over what goes into your food and helps you manage your calorie intake without sacrificing flavor. Here are some cooking techniques that can help you keep calories in check while still delivering delicious, satisfying meals:

- **Grilling and Baking**: Grilling and baking are great alternatives to frying, as they require less oil. You can still get those delicious crispy textures—try grilling chicken breast or baking your potatoes instead of frying them.

- **Air Frying**: As mentioned earlier, air frying is a fantastic way to get that crispy, fried flavor without the oil and added calories of deep frying. You can use it for chicken, fries, vegetables, or even reheating leftovers to maintain crispiness.

- **Marinating**: Instead of using heavy sauces or breading, try marinating your meats and vegetables in flavorful mixtures made with herbs, spices, and a small amount of healthy fat like olive oil. Marinating adds lots of flavor without excess calories.

- **Using Spices and Herbs**: One of the best ways to add flavor to your meals without adding calories is by using a variety of spices and herbs. Garlic, ginger, cumin, paprika, basil, thyme—these are just a few examples of how you can make a simple dish taste like it came from a gourmet restaurant.

- **Lower-Calorie Swaps**: There are so many ways to modify recipes to make them lower in calories while still keeping them tasty. Greek yogurt can replace sour cream, applesauce can be used in place of oil in baking, and cauliflower rice is a great substitute for traditional rice.

3.6 Understanding Portion Control and Listening to Your Body

Crafting a balanced plate isn't just about choosing the right foods—it's also about knowing how much of each food to eat. **Portion control** is crucial when you're trying to lose weight, but it doesn't have to mean tiny, unsatisfying meals. It's about understanding how to portion foods to get the most volume and satisfaction within your calorie goals.

- **Portioning Carbs and Fats**: Carbs and fats are more calorie-dense than protein and vegetables, so controlling portions of these components is key. For example, a serving of pasta is typically about half a cup cooked—far less than most people serve themselves. Instead of filling half your plate with pasta, try combining it with spiralized zucchini to add volume without the extra calories.

- **Volume Eating with Vegetables**: Vegetables are low in calories and high in fiber, making them perfect for adding volume to your meals. You can fill half your plate with veggies and still be well within your calorie target. Eating a large volume of vegetables helps you feel full, which makes sticking to a calorie deficit much easier.

- **Mindful Eating**: One of the best ways to manage portion sizes without feeling restricted is by practicing **mindful eating**. Eat slowly, chew thoroughly, and truly taste your food. Pay attention to how your body feels as you eat—are you still hungry, or are you satisfied? Often, we eat past the point of satisfaction out of habit or because the food tastes good. Learning to identify your body's cues and stop eating when you're full can help you enjoy all foods in moderation.

3.7 Making Meals at Home: Recipes to Fit Your Goals

Cooking at home allows you to customize meals to fit your calorie and nutrient needs while keeping them enjoyable. Here are a few recipe ideas to try:

- **Air Fryer Fried Chicken**: Enjoy crispy, seasoned chicken without all the oil. Coat chicken pieces in a mixture of seasoned panko breadcrumbs or crushed cornflakes, spray with a little cooking oil, and air fry until crispy and cooked through. Serve with a side of roasted veggies and a small serving of mashed potatoes.

- **Loaded Turkey Burger Bowl**: Skip the bun and make a burger bowl with a lean turkey patty, lots of greens, roasted sweet potatoes, cherry tomatoes, cucumber, and a drizzle of light ranch or yogurt-based dressing. You get all the flavors of a burger with fewer calories and more nutrients.

- **Sheet Pan Fajitas**: Slice chicken breast, bell peppers, and onions, and season with chili powder, paprika, cumin, and a bit of olive oil. Spread everything on a sheet pan and bake until the chicken is cooked through and the veggies are tender. Serve with whole-wheat tortillas or lettuce wraps, and top with salsa, a bit of cheese, and Greek yogurt.

3.8 Planning Ahead: Creating a Weekly Meal Blueprint

Planning ahead can make it much easier to consistently craft balanced plates throughout the week. Here are some strategies to create a flexible meal plan that helps you stay on track:

- **Create a Meal Template**: Instead of planning every single meal in detail, create a simple template that you can adjust based on your preferences. For example:

  - **Breakfast**: A protein (like eggs or Greek yogurt) + a carbohydrate (like oats or whole-grain toast) + a fruit.

  - **Lunch**: A lean protein (like chicken or tofu) + lots of non-starchy veggies + a carbohydrate (like quinoa or sweet potato).

  - **Dinner**: A protein (like fish or lean beef) + a large portion of veggies + healthy fats (like avocado or nuts).

- **Batch Prep Components**: Prepare components of your meals ahead of time so that putting a balanced plate together is quick and easy. Cook grains, roast veggies, and marinate proteins on the weekend so that all you need to do is assemble them into meals throughout the week.

- **Stay Flexible**: Life happens, and plans can change. If you don't feel like eating what you planned, use your stocked kitchen to create something that still fits your template. Flexibility is key to making sure you can stay consistent over time.

3.9 Eating Out and Balancing Indulgence

Eating out is often seen as a challenge when trying to lose weight, but it doesn't have to be. You can still enjoy meals at your favorite restaurants if you apply the principles of balance and portion control.

- **Choose Protein and Veggies**: Look for options that have a good source of protein and vegetables. For example, opt for grilled chicken and vegetables instead of fried options, or ask for extra veggies instead of fries.

- **Watch Portions**: Restaurant portions are often much larger than what you would serve yourself at home. Consider splitting an entree with someone, or immediately ask for a to-go box and put half of your meal away before you start eating.

- **Focus on Enjoyment**: Eating out is also about enjoying the experience. Choose foods you genuinely want to eat and savor them. Eating slowly and mindfully not only enhances your enjoyment but also makes it easier to recognize when you're satisfied.

3.10 Conclusion: Mastering the Balanced Plate for Sustainable Weight Loss

Crafting a balanced plate isn't just about losing weight; it's about learning how to nourish your body while also enjoying the foods you love. When you learn to incorporate all the elements—protein, healthy fats, carbohydrates, and fiber—you build meals that are satisfying, nutritious, and perfectly tailored to your goals.

Remember that a balanced plate allows room for the foods you crave. It's not about eliminating indulgences; it's about making them work within your overall diet in a way that helps you feel great, stay on track, and reach your goals. This chapter gives you the blueprint for success—a way to lose weight while enjoying every bite along the journey.

Chapter 4: How to Eat at Restaurants and Social Events Without Going Off Track

4.1 The Challenge of Eating Out: Overcoming Fear and Guilt

Eating out can be daunting for many people trying to lose weight. Restaurants often serve dishes loaded with hidden calories—extra butter, sauces, oils, and portion sizes that are significantly larger than what we'd serve ourselves at home. Add in peer pressure and social expectations, and it's no wonder people often feel their progress is threatened every time they step into a restaurant or attend a social event.

Yet eating out and socializing are parts of life that can—and should—be enjoyed without guilt. This chapter will help you develop strategies to confidently eat out, allowing you to take part in life's pleasures while staying on track with your health goals. Whether it's an upscale restaurant, a casual diner, or a friend's barbecue, the key to maintaining progress lies in preparation, smart choices, and a balanced mindset.

4.2 Shifting Your Mindset: From Fear to Freedom

Before diving into specific strategies, it's crucial to address the mindset required to successfully navigate eating out. The key to enjoying eating out without going off track is letting go of perfectionism and embracing **flexibility**.

- **Food Is More Than Fuel**: Eating is more than just fueling your body. It's a social, emotional, and even cultural experience that brings people together. Instead of fearing the food served at restaurants or social events, try to appreciate the experience for what it is—an opportunity to connect with others and enjoy the atmosphere. It's about being present in the moment, rather than focusing solely on calorie counts.

- **Avoiding All-Or-Nothing Thinking**: One of the biggest challenges is avoiding all-or-nothing thinking. Many people think if they've had one high-calorie item, they've "ruined" the day and may as well overeat for the rest of it. This kind of thinking can set back progress and make it difficult to stay consistent. Instead, focus on **balance**—one indulgent meal doesn't undo all your progress, and it's okay to enjoy yourself without overindulging.

- **Mindful Eating and Enjoyment**: Mindful eating is particularly useful when eating out. This involves savoring each bite, eating slowly, and being fully aware of the experience. This helps not only with enjoying your food more but also recognizing when you're full, which prevents overeating. You'll be surprised how much satisfaction can come from eating consciously and appreciating each bite.

4.3 Planning Ahead: Setting Yourself Up for Success

When eating out, planning ahead can make all the difference in making smart choices without feeling overwhelmed. This part of the chapter covers how to prepare before even stepping into the restaurant.

- **Look at Menus in Advance**: Many restaurants now have their menus available online, often with nutritional information included. Spend a few minutes looking over the menu before you go, especially if you know that spontaneity often leads to choosing the less optimal options. Deciding what to eat beforehand helps reduce the pressure to make a quick choice under social influence, which can make you more susceptible to ordering calorie-heavy dishes.

- **Have a Calorie Goal in Mind**: Knowing your calorie goal for the day can help guide your choices. If you're planning on indulging a bit, try to adjust your intake earlier in the day—opt for lighter meals that are high in protein and vegetables, keeping your calorie count lower so you can accommodate for a more indulgent evening.

- **Avoid Arriving Overly Hungry**: Going to a restaurant when you're starving is a recipe for overeating. If you're too hungry, you're more likely to make impulsive choices and overeat once the food arrives. Have a small snack—such as a piece of fruit, a handful of nuts, or some yogurt—before you go to take the edge off your hunger.

4.4 Reading the Menu: Identifying Hidden Calorie Bombs

Restaurant menus are designed to entice, often using descriptive words like "crispy," "creamy," or "buttery" to make items sound irresistible. Being able to decipher menu language is key to making informed decisions.

- **Keywords to Look For:**

  - **Avoid** dishes described as **fried, creamy, smothered, crispy, battered, breaded, cheesy**, or **rich**, as these are often loaded with extra fats and calories.

  - **Opt for** dishes described as **grilled, baked, broiled, steamed, roasted**, or **poached**. These cooking methods tend to use less oil, reducing the calorie content.

- **Watch the Sides**: Pay attention to the side dishes. Many entrees come with calorie-dense sides like fries, mashed potatoes, or pasta. Ask if you can substitute these for a side salad, steamed vegetables, or another lighter option. This simple swap can save hundreds of calories.

- **Check for Hidden Fats and Sugars**: Sauces and dressings can contain hidden sugars and fats that add up quickly. If you're ordering a salad, ask for the dressing on the side, and consider dipping your fork in the dressing before taking a bite rather than pouring it all over. For main dishes, request that heavy sauces be served on the side so you can control the amount.

4.5 Portion Control: How to Handle Oversized Servings

Restaurant portions are often much larger than what you would typically serve yourself at home. To avoid overeating, employ these portion control strategies:

- **Split an Entree**: If you're dining with someone else, consider splitting an entree. Many restaurant portions are large enough for two people. By sharing, you can enjoy the meal without consuming the full calorie load.

- **Ask for a To-Go Box Early**: If splitting isn't an option, ask for a to-go box when your food arrives and immediately put half of it away. This can prevent you from mindlessly finishing your entire plate simply because it's there. You'll not only save calories but also have a delicious meal for later.

- **Start with a Salad or Soup**: Starting with a broth-based soup or a garden salad (with dressing on the side) can help fill you up before your main course arrives. The fiber in vegetables or the volume from soup can curb your appetite, reducing the chances of overeating the more calorie-dense main dish.

- **Eat Slowly and Mindfully**: Eating slowly gives your brain time to register that you're full, which takes about 20 minutes. When dining out, take your time—engage in conversation, put your fork down between bites, and savor each bite. This will help you eat less and enjoy your meal more.

4.6 Specific Cuisine Strategies: Navigating Common Restaurants

Different types of cuisine present different challenges, so here are some tips for making smarter choices at popular types of restaurants:

- **Italian Restaurants:**

  - **Choose Wisely:** Italian menus are often filled with high-calorie pasta dishes and cream-based sauces. Opt for dishes like **grilled chicken or fish with vegetables,** or **pasta with marinara sauce** rather than Alfredo.

  - **Control Portions:** Italian portions can be very large, especially when it comes to pasta. Consider ordering an appetizer-sized portion, or ask for half to be packed up before you start eating.

- **Mexican Restaurants:**

  - **Focus on Lean Proteins:** Look for **fajitas** (chicken or shrimp), **grilled fish tacos,** or **chicken burritos** without cheese or sour cream.

  - **Be Careful with the Chips:** Chips and salsa are often put on the table as soon as you sit down. If you want to indulge, set a limit—perhaps 5 or 10 chips—rather than mindlessly eating through the entire basket.

- **Asian Restaurants:**

o **Chinese Cuisine**: Many Chinese dishes are high in calories due to frying and sugary sauces. Opt for **steamed chicken and vegetables, stir-fries with light sauce, or hot and sour soup.**

o **Japanese Cuisine**: Sushi can be a great choice, but beware of rolls with cream cheese, tempura, or mayo-based sauces. Stick to **sashimi, nigiri, or basic rolls** without the extras, and enjoy **edamame or miso soup** as a starter.

- **American Steakhouses:**

o **Choose Lean Meats**: Opt for **leaner cuts** like **filet mignon** or **sirloin**, and pair them with a **side of steamed vegetables** or **a side salad.**

o **Avoid Calorie-Dense Sides**: Sides like **loaded mashed potatoes** and **creamed spinach** can be high in calories. Opt for **baked potatoes without butter, green beans,** or **roasted asparagus** instead.

- **Brunch or Breakfast Restaurants:**

o **Choose Protein-Rich Options**: Look for items like **scrambled eggs, omelets with**

veggies, or **Greek yogurt with fruit**. Avoid dishes like **French toast, pancakes with syrup**, or **loaded breakfast burritos**, which can be very high in calories.

- **Customize Your Order**: Ask for egg dishes to be **cooked with minimal oil or butter**, and request **whole-grain toast** rather than white. Opt for **fruit** instead of hash browns as a side.

4.7 Alcohol: Navigating Drinks at Restaurants and Social Gatherings

Alcohol is often present at social gatherings and restaurants, and it can easily add a significant amount of empty calories to your daily intake. However, you can still enjoy a drink if you approach it mindfully.

- **Stick to Clear Spirits**: Clear spirits like **vodka, gin, or tequila** mixed with **soda water** and a splash of citrus are lower-calorie options compared to sugary cocktails. Avoid drinks like **margaritas, piña coladas**, or **sweet liqueurs**, which are often loaded with sugar.

- **Choose Light Beer or Wine: Light beer** and **dry wine** (white or red) are also reasonable choices if you prefer something other than hard liquor. Just be mindful of portion sizes—alcoholic drinks can quickly add up in calories.

- **Avoid Sugary Mixers**: Many cocktails come with high-calorie mixers like **fruit juices, syrups**, or **cola**.

Ask for alternatives like **diet soda, soda water**, or **light juice.**

- **Set a Limit and Hydrate**: Alcohol can also lower inhibitions, making it harder to stick to your calorie goals. Set a limit on how many drinks you'll have before going out, and alternate between alcoholic drinks and water to stay hydrated and slow down your alcohol intake.

4.8 Social Events: Potlucks, Buffets, and Family Gatherings

Social events like buffets, potlucks, and family gatherings can be particularly challenging because you often have less control over the food that's available. Here are some tips to navigate these situations:

- **Bring Your Own Dish**: If it's a potluck, bring a dish that fits your goals. This ensures there's at least one option available that you know is aligned with your eating plan. Consider a **large salad, roasted vegetables**, or **a lean protein dish.**

- **Survey Before Serving**: At a buffet, do a walkthrough before filling your plate. Take stock of all the options available, and then decide what you really want. Aim to fill your plate mostly with **lean proteins and vegetables**, saving a smaller portion for any indulgent options you'd like to try.

- **Use a Small Plate**: If possible, use a smaller plate. This helps you manage portions by physically limiting how much you can serve yourself in one go.

- **Prioritize Protein and Vegetables**: Fill up on protein-rich items like **grilled chicken, fish, or beans** and vegetables first. These foods will help keep you satisfied without overeating high-calorie options.

- **Mindful Eating**: It can be easy to overeat in a social setting when you're distracted. Practice mindful eating—sit down while you eat, chew thoroughly, and savor each bite. This helps you notice when you're full and prevents you from eating just because food is available.

4.9 Handling Peer Pressure and Social Expectations

Family and friends often have good intentions, but they may not fully understand your goals, which can lead to unwanted pressure to eat more or indulge beyond what you feel comfortable with. Here's how to navigate these social dynamics:

- **Practice Saying No Politely**: It's okay to say no. Be polite but firm—something like, "No thank you, I'm full," or "I'm trying to make healthier choices" is enough. Most people will respect your decision if you're clear about it.

- **Have a Plan**: If you know that Aunt Mary always insists you try her pie, plan ahead. Decide if you'll have a small slice or politely decline. Having a plan reduces the stress of being put on the spot.

- **Use Non-Food-Based Compliments**: Often, people push food because they want validation. If someone offers you their homemade dish and you don't want to eat it, try complimenting them in a different way. For instance, say, "That looks amazing, you're such a great cook!" This acknowledges their effort without having to eat more than you want.

- **Eat Before You Go**: If you're worried about not having enough options, eat a healthy, filling meal before attending the event. This way, you're less likely to be hungry and can make better choices once you arrive.

4.10 The Importance of Hydration During Social Events

Hydration is a crucial but often overlooked part of managing calorie intake during social events. Dehydration can sometimes be mistaken for hunger, leading to unnecessary eating.

- **Drink Water Before Eating**: Having a glass of water before eating can help you feel fuller and prevent overeating. Keep a glass of water with you throughout the event and take sips regularly.

- **Avoid Sugary Drinks**: Sugar-laden beverages like **punches, sweetened iced teas, or sodas** can add a lot of empty calories without filling you up. Stick to **water, sparkling water**, or **diet drinks**. This allows you to save those calories for food that will actually satisfy you.

4.11 Celebrating Small Victories and Learning from Setbacks

Successfully navigating a social event or dining out while sticking to your goals is an accomplishment worth celebrating. These small wins build confidence and help you establish healthy habits that will support long-term success.

- **Celebrate Your Wins**: Whether it's resisting the urge to overeat at a buffet, making a healthier choice at a restaurant, or simply enjoying your meal mindfully, these are all wins that should be acknowledged. Treat yourself in non-food ways—like buying a book you've wanted, having a relaxing spa day, or just giving yourself some well-deserved downtime.

- **Learn from Setbacks**: Setbacks are part of the journey, and they happen to everyone. If you overeat or make a choice you're unhappy with, reflect on what happened and how you felt. What triggered that choice? How can you make a different decision next time? Treat every setback as a learning opportunity and move forward with more knowledge and experience.

4.12 Summary: Making Dining Out and Social Events Work for You

Dining out and attending social events are integral parts of life, and they should be enjoyed—not feared. By shifting your mindset, planning ahead, making strategic choices, and learning to handle social pressures, you can stay on track with your weight loss goals while still enjoying the experience.

The key takeaway from this chapter is that successful weight management isn't about avoiding these events—it's about learning how to navigate them in a way that fits your goals. With practice, you'll find it becomes easier and more natural to make choices that align with your health journey, allowing you to savor both the food and the moments spent with family and friends.

5.1 The Power of Small Changes: Why Smart Swaps Matter

5.1.1 Weight Loss Without Deprivation

One of the most common reasons people struggle with weight loss is that many diets require you to give up the foods you love. The key problem with restrictive diets is that they often lead to feelings of deprivation, which in turn can cause you to give up entirely or binge on the very foods you're trying to avoid. Smart swaps offer a solution: they allow you to continue enjoying the flavors and textures you love while making minor adjustments to reduce calories, unhealthy fats, or added sugars. Over time, these small changes add up, making weight loss sustainable and attainable without making life miserable.

The goal of smart swaps is to replace high-calorie, low-nutrient items with options that offer more nutritional benefits and fewer empty calories. By choosing foods that are rich in vitamins, minerals, and macronutrients like protein and fiber, you not only support weight loss but also improve your energy levels, digestion, and overall health.

5.1.2 Building a New Relationship with Food

Food should be nourishing, satisfying, and enjoyable. Too often, weight loss goals create a sense of anxiety around food choices—people feel guilty for eating something "bad" or feel restricted because they can't have something they want. Smart swaps aim to change that relationship by encouraging mindful choices that align with your goals without creating a sense of loss. For example, choosing a leaner protein, a different type of grain, or a lower-sugar version of your favorite treat allows you to stay on track while still enjoying the experience of eating.

Instead of thinking about what you "can't have," smart swaps focus on what you can enjoy. They give you more control, more options, and more room to explore flavors and ingredients, transforming your diet into something sustainable rather than a temporary fix.

5.2 Smart Swaps for Breakfast: Starting Your Day with the Right Choices

5.2.1 Understanding Breakfast's Impact on Weight Loss

Breakfast is often said to "set the tone" for the rest of the day. A balanced, nutrient-rich breakfast can help regulate blood sugar levels, reduce hunger later in the day, and set you up for success. The key to smart swaps at breakfast is balancing protein, healthy fats, and fiber to create a meal that is filling and energizing without excessive calories.

5.2.2 Reducing Empty Calories: Swaps for Popular Breakfast Foods

- **Sugary Cereals vs. Whole-Grain Alternatives:** Many breakfast cereals are marketed as healthy but are often full of added sugars and refined carbohydrates, leading to a rapid spike and drop in blood sugar. Rolled oats, steel-cut oats, or whole-grain bran cereals are fantastic alternatives that provide slow-releasing energy. To add flavor without added sugar, you can mix in cinnamon, a teaspoon of honey, or fresh fruit.

- **Pastries vs. Protein-Rich Options:** Pastries like croissants, muffins, or doughnuts are high in refined carbs, sugars, and fats. A better option is whole-grain toast with nut butter or Greek yogurt with a handful of berries and some nuts. These swaps introduce protein and healthy fats, which contribute to satiety and prevent the mid-morning crash that often follows a sugary breakfast.

- **Pancakes and Syrup vs. Banana Pancakes:** Traditional pancakes made with white flour and topped with sugary syrup can be high in calories and lacking in nutritional value. Instead, try banana pancakes made with just eggs, mashed bananas, and a little cinnamon. They're lower in calories, have no refined sugars, and include more protein. Add a drizzle of pure maple syrup or a handful of fresh berries for sweetness.

5.2.3 Spotlight on Protein: The Key to a Satisfying Breakfast

Protein is crucial for keeping hunger at bay, especially in the morning. By adding more protein to your breakfast, you not only make the meal more satisfying but also reduce the likelihood of overeating later.

- **Swap Sugary Yogurts for Greek Yogurt:** Greek yogurt is a much better option than many flavored yogurts, which can be loaded with sugar. Greek yogurt has significantly more protein and provides a creamy texture without the need for added sugar. If you crave sweetness, add fresh berries, a small drizzle of honey, or a sprinkle of nuts and seeds.

- **Egg Muffins vs. Bagels:** Instead of having a high-calorie bagel topped with cream cheese, consider making egg muffins baked with vegetables, a sprinkle of cheese, and lean protein like turkey sausage. These muffins are portable, easy to prepare in advance, and provide a protein-rich, lower-calorie start to your day.

5.2.4 Balancing Fats: Healthy Swaps for Breakfast Fats

- **Butter vs. Avocado or Nut Butter:** While butter is often used as a spread on toast, it is high in saturated fats. Replacing it with avocado or nut butter not only cuts down on unhealthy fats but also introduces healthy monounsaturated fats, which help keep you full. Avocado toast with a sprinkle of sea salt and red pepper flakes is a simple, nutrient-packed way to start your day.

- **Cooking Oils vs. Non-Stick Spray:** If you're frying eggs or vegetables, consider using a non-stick spray or a small amount of olive oil rather than a large dollop of butter. This can save up to 100 calories per meal while still providing enough fat for cooking.

5.3 Smart Swaps for Lunch: Crafting a Balanced, Satisfying Midday Meal

5.3.1 Common Lunch Pitfalls and How to Overcome Them

Lunch is a pivotal meal for maintaining energy levels throughout the day. However, many lunch options—whether from home or the office cafeteria—tend to be high in refined carbs, fats, or added sugars, which can lead to an afternoon slump. The key is to create a lunch that balances protein, fiber, and healthy fats, providing sustained energy without excessive calories.

5.3.2 Sandwich Makeover: Bread, Spreads, and Fillings

- **Bread Choices:** Instead of white bread, which is often stripped of fiber and nutrients, opt for whole-grain bread, Ezekiel bread, or whole-wheat wraps. These alternatives have a lower glycemic index, which helps prevent a sharp rise in blood sugar, and they provide more fiber to keep you full longer.

- **Spreads:** Mayo can add a surprising number of calories to a sandwich. Replacing mayonnaise with mustard, avocado, or a Greek yogurt-based spread can significantly cut down on calories while boosting nutrients. You can also make your own flavorful spread by mixing Greek yogurt with herbs, garlic, and a little lemon juice.

- **Fillings:** Instead of processed deli meats (which can be high in sodium and preservatives), choose lean proteins like grilled chicken, turkey, or tuna. You can also make vegetarian sandwiches with hummus, grilled veggies, or tofu for a lower-calorie and nutrient-dense option.

5.3.3 Salad Enhancements: Avoiding Hidden Calories

Salads can either be a very healthy choice or a calorie trap depending on the ingredients. Here are some swaps to keep your salads healthy and satisfying:

- **Dressing:** Salad dressings can add a large number of unnecessary calories, especially creamy dressings like ranch or blue cheese. Swap these for vinaigrettes made with olive oil and vinegar, or even salsa or Greek yogurt-based dressings. Always ask for your dressing on the side so you can control how much you use.

- **Croutons:** Croutons are usually fried and high in empty carbs. Replace them with toasted nuts or seeds for a crunchy texture. This adds healthy fats and protein instead of empty calories.

- **Cheese:** If you love cheese, opt for a small amount of a strong-flavored cheese like feta or parmesan. These cheeses pack a lot of flavor, so you can use less and still get the taste, reducing the overall calories of your salad.

5.3.4 Grain-Based Lunches: Healthier Alternatives

Many lunches are built around grains, like rice or pasta. Here are some swaps that allow you to still enjoy these meals while keeping the calories in check:

5.3.4 Grain-Based Lunches: Healthier Alternatives (continued)

- **Pasta vs. Legume Pasta:** Traditional pasta can be calorie-dense and not very filling due to its lack of fiber and protein. **Legume-based pastas** made from lentils, chickpeas, or black beans are excellent alternatives. They are higher in protein and fiber, helping to keep you full for longer and providing more nutrients. Plus, they still have that chewy pasta texture that you love. Another option is **whole wheat pasta**, which is slightly higher in fiber compared to white pasta and has a lower glycemic index, helping stabilize your blood sugar.

- **Regular Couscous vs. Whole Grain Couscous or Farro**: If you enjoy couscous, try swapping **regular couscous** with **whole grain couscous** or **farro**. These options have more fiber and a lower glycemic index. **Farro** has a chewy texture and a nutty flavor, making it a great addition to salads, bowls, or as a side dish.

- **Noodles vs. Shirataki Noodles**: If you're looking for a low-calorie alternative to noodles, **shirataki noodles** are a fantastic option. Made from konjac yam, they are extremely low in calories and provide a similar texture to traditional noodles. They are perfect for stir-fries, pasta dishes, and soups where you want to enjoy a generous portion without the calories.

5.3.5 Wraps and Bowls: Making Every Ingredient Count

- **Tortilla Wraps vs. Lettuce Wraps**: Wraps are a popular choice for lunch, but they can sometimes contain more calories than expected, especially if they're made with **white flour tortillas**. Swapping a **tortilla** for **lettuce wraps** or **collard green wraps** provides a crunchy texture, keeps calories low, and significantly boosts the nutrient content. You could also choose **low-carb or whole wheat tortillas** for fewer calories compared to regular ones.

- **Burrito Bowls with Smart Substitutions**: Burrito bowls can be calorie-heavy, but by making a few substitutions, you can create a balanced, lighter meal. Swap **white rice** for **cauliflower rice**, choose **lean proteins** like **grilled chicken or shrimp** instead of ground beef, and use **Greek yogurt** instead of sour cream. Pile on fresh vegetables like **tomatoes, bell peppers**, and **greens** for volume and fiber.

- **Wrap Fillings**: Instead of filling your wrap with **breaded chicken**, opt for **grilled chicken breast, tofu**, or **black beans** for a protein-rich option. You can add **avocado** for healthy fats and **hummus** for creaminess without relying on calorie-dense cheeses or mayonnaise. Adding plenty of crunchy vegetables like **cucumbers, bell peppers**, and **carrots** keeps the wrap filling and adds texture.

5.3.6 Soups as a Filling Lunch Option

- **Creamy Soups vs. Broth-Based or Blended Veggie Soups**: Creamy soups, such as **clam chowder** or **broccoli cheddar**, are typically made with heavy cream and butter, which means they can be high in calories. Instead, opt for **broth-based soups** or **blended vegetable soups**. Soups like **minestrone, chicken vegetable, lentil**, or **butternut squash** are satisfying, lower in calories, and packed with nutrients.

- **Adding Beans and Vegetables for Volume**: If you enjoy a particular soup but want to make it more filling and reduce calorie density, consider adding **vegetables and legumes**. Adding **zucchini, carrots, spinach**, or **beans** can increase the volume, making the soup more satisfying without adding a lot of calories.

- **Homemade Soups vs. Canned Soups**: Store-bought canned soups can be loaded with sodium and preservatives. Making **homemade soup** allows you to control the ingredients, reduce the sodium content, and add plenty of nutrient-rich vegetables and lean proteins. Preparing a large batch on the weekend and storing portions in the fridge or freezer makes for an easy, healthy lunch option during the week.

5.4 Smart Swaps for Dinner: Keeping Your Evening Meal Light Yet Satisfying

5.4.1 Dinner Pitfalls: Why Evening Meals Can Be Calorie Traps

Dinner is often the time when many people relax after a long day, and food choices can be influenced by convenience, fatigue, or a desire for comfort. Unfortunately, this can lead to calorie-heavy dinners that are difficult to digest before bedtime, affecting sleep quality and potentially leading to weight gain. Making smart swaps helps keep dinners balanced and nutrient-dense without sacrificing flavor or comfort.

5.4.2 Smart Protein Swaps for Dinner

- **Fried Proteins vs. Grilled or Baked**: Fried meats, like **fried chicken or battered fish**, can add hundreds of extra calories due to the cooking oil. Instead, bake or grill your protein to keep the flavors intact without all the additional calories. For instance, make **oven-baked "fried" chicken** by coating the chicken in seasoned panko breadcrumbs and baking it until crispy.

- **Red Meat vs. Leaner Proteins**: Red meat, such as **beef and lamb**, is higher in saturated fats and calories compared to leaner proteins like **chicken breast, turkey**, or **white fish**. Swapping **ground beef** for **ground turkey** or **chicken** in dishes like tacos, meatloaf, or burgers significantly reduces calories and fat while still providing a delicious and satisfying meal.

- **Plant-Based Proteins**: Incorporate **tofu, tempeh, beans, lentils**, or **legume-based protein crumbles** for a lighter option. They are not only lower in fat but also rich in fiber, which helps keep you full. **Black bean burgers** or **chickpea patties** are great alternatives to traditional beef burgers.

5.4.3 Swapping Out Calorie-Dense Side Dishes

- **Mashed Potatoes vs. Mashed Cauliflower or Root Vegetables**: Traditional mashed potatoes made with **butter and cream** can be high in calories. Instead, opt for **mashed cauliflower, turnips**, or a blend of **root vegetables**. These swaps maintain the creamy texture but with far fewer calories. You can also add roasted garlic or herbs like thyme and rosemary for added flavor.

- **Pasta vs. Spiralized Vegetables**: Traditional pasta can be very calorie-dense, especially when topped with creamy sauces. Instead, try **zoodles (zucchini noodles), carrot noodles**, or **spaghetti squash**. These vegetable-based alternatives are significantly lower in calories and carbs, while still providing the satisfaction of twirling your fork into a "pasta" dish.

- **Rice vs. Quinoa, Barley, or Cauliflower Rice**: Swap **white rice** for **whole grains** like **quinoa** or **barley**, which are higher in fiber and protein. If you want to cut down on carbs even further, **cauliflower rice** is a great option. It's low in calories, cooks quickly, and can easily take on the flavors of the dish.

5.4.4 Making Vegetables the Star of Your Plate

Vegetables are often thought of as side dishes, but they can easily be transformed into the main part of your meal. By incorporating more vegetables into your dinner, you can significantly reduce calorie density while still enjoying a hearty, satisfying meal.

- **Stuffed Vegetables**: Instead of making a meat-heavy dish, try **stuffing vegetables** like **bell peppers, zucchini, or eggplant**. Fill them with a mix of **lean protein (ground turkey or lentils), quinoa**, and **spices** for a hearty, flavorful dinner that's lower in calories and higher in fiber.

- **Vegetable-Based Casseroles**: Traditional casseroles can be heavy on cheese, cream, and processed carbs. Instead, make **vegetable-based casseroles** like **eggplant lasagna** (using eggplant slices instead of pasta) or **zucchini and mushroom gratin** with a light sprinkling of cheese. These dishes are comforting but won't weigh you down.

- **Cauliflower Steaks**: Replace a traditional meat steak with a **roasted cauliflower steak** marinated with herbs and spices. While it won't be exactly like a beef steak, it offers a satisfying texture and is a fantastic way to keep the meal lower in calories. Pair it with a side of **whole grains** and a **yogurt-based sauce**.

5.4.5 Sauces, Dressings, and Seasonings: Reducing Hidden Calories

- **Creamy Sauces vs. Yogurt or Vegetable-Based Sauces**: Creamy sauces like Alfredo or cheese sauce can add a large number of calories and fat to an otherwise balanced dish. Instead, use **Greek yogurt** as a base for a lighter cream sauce or make a **pureed vegetable sauce** with **roasted red peppers, tomatoes,** or **butternut squash**. These options add creaminess and flavor without all the excess calories.

- **Butter vs. Olive Oil or Ghee**: Instead of butter, consider using **extra virgin olive oil** or **ghee** in moderation. **Olive oil** contains healthy fats and has anti-inflammatory properties, while **ghee** has a rich flavor and is easier to digest for some people compared to butter. Using a small amount of these fats allows you to enjoy rich flavors without overdoing it.

- **Store-Bought Marinades vs. Homemade Marinades**: Pre-made marinades can be high in sugar and sodium. Make your own marinades using **citrus juice (like lemon or lime), herbs, spices, garlic**, and **a little olive oil**. Homemade marinades not only taste fresher but also allow you to control the ingredients, keeping the calorie count lower.

5.4.6 Smart Cooking Techniques for Lighter Dinners

- **Roasting Instead of Frying**: Roasting vegetables and proteins instead of frying significantly reduces calories while maintaining flavor. **Roasting** brings out the natural sweetness in vegetables and creates a caramelized texture, making them a great addition to any meal.

- **Steaming Instead of Boiling**: Steaming vegetables helps retain their nutrients compared to boiling, where many nutrients can be lost in the cooking water. Steamed vegetables can be seasoned with **fresh herbs, lemon zest,** or **a sprinkle of nutritional yeast** to add flavor without excess calories.

- **Air Frying for Texture:** An **air fryer** can replicate the crispiness of fried foods without the need for large amounts of oil. You can make **crispy chicken strips, vegetable fritters,** or even **homemade fries** using the air fryer for a fraction of the calories compared to deep frying.

5.5 Smart Swaps for Snacks and Desserts: Enjoying Treats Without the Guilt

5.5.1 Snacking with Purpose: Making Snacks Nutrient-Dense

Snacks can be one of the biggest sources of unnecessary calories, especially if you're reaching for **processed options** like chips, cookies, or candy. Making smart swaps in your snacks can help you stay on track and feel more satisfied between meals.

- **Potato Chips vs. Veggie Chips or Popcorn: Potato chips** are high in fat and calories, with little nutritional value. Instead, opt for **veggie chips** (like kale chips or beet chips) made with minimal oil. You can also air-pop **popcorn** and season it with **nutritional yeast, paprika,** or **cinnamon** for a light and flavorful snack.

- **Candy Bars vs. Dark Chocolate and Nuts:** Candy bars are often loaded with sugars, unhealthy fats, and artificial ingredients. Swap them for **a piece of dark chocolate (70% cocoa or higher)** paired with **a handful of nuts.** This combination still provides the sweet and rich flavor you crave but with far less sugar and added healthy fats and protein to keep you fuller longer.

- **Pretzels vs. Raw Veggies and Hummus**: Pretzels may seem like a light snack, but they're often high in refined carbs and sodium without much nutritional value. Swap pretzels for **carrot sticks, cucumber slices**, or **bell pepper strips** dipped in **hummus**. The veggies add fiber, and the hummus provides protein and healthy fats, making for a more balanced and satisfying snack.

- **Granola Bars vs. Homemade Energy Bites**: Store-bought granola bars can be packed with added sugars and preservatives. Instead, make **homemade energy bites** with **oats, nut butter, honey**, and **cacao nibs**. These bites are easy to prepare, portable, and allow you to control the ingredients.

5.5.2 Desserts with Less Guilt: Healthier Treat Alternatives

- **Ice Cream vs. Frozen Greek Yogurt or "Nice Cream"**: Traditional ice cream is high in sugar and fat, which can add up quickly if you're having it regularly. Swap it for **frozen Greek yogurt** with **fresh fruit** or make **banana "nice cream"** by blending frozen bananas with a little **vanilla extract** and **a splash of**

almond milk. This creates a creamy, delicious treat without all the added sugars.

- **Cookies vs. Oatmeal Cookies or Fruit-Based Treats**: Instead of traditional sugar-laden cookies, make **oatmeal cookies** with **rolled oats, mashed banana,** and **a handful of dark chocolate chips**. Another option is **baked apples** with **cinnamon and a drizzle of honey**, which gives you the sweet, warm flavor you crave in a dessert with fewer calories and more fiber.

- **Cheesecake vs. Greek Yogurt Parfait**: Cheesecake can be very calorie-dense, with lots of added sugar and fat. Instead, make a **Greek yogurt parfait** by layering **Greek yogurt** with **fresh berries, granola,** and a drizzle of **honey**. It's creamy, rich, and satisfying but with far fewer calories and much more protein.

- **Chocolate Pudding vs. Avocado Chocolate Mousse**: Traditional chocolate pudding is often high in sugar and contains additives. **Avocado chocolate mousse** is a great alternative that's creamy and indulgent without all the added sugar. Blend **ripe avocado** with **cocoa powder, a bit of honey or agave,** and **vanilla extract** for a healthier dessert option rich in healthy fats.

5.6 Smart Swaps for Drinks: Reducing Liquid Calories

5.6.1 The Hidden Danger of Liquid Calories

Many people underestimate how many calories they consume in beverages. Sugary sodas, juices, fancy coffee drinks, and alcoholic beverages can all add significant calories without providing much nutritional value or satiety. By making smart swaps, you can save hundreds of calories each day.

5.6.2 Smart Swaps for Common High-Calorie Drinks

- **Sugary Soda vs. Diet Soda or Sparkling Water:** **Sugary sodas** are one of the biggest contributors to empty calorie intake. Instead, switch to **diet soda**, which contains no sugar, or opt for **sparkling water**. You can add a splash of **100% fruit juice** or fresh fruit slices like **lemon, lime**, or **berries** for flavor without adding many calories.

- **Fruit Juice vs. Infused Water or Herbal Tea**: While **fruit juice** may seem healthy, it often contains as much sugar as soda. Replace juice with **infused water** (like cucumber or strawberry mint water) or **unsweetened herbal tea**. These options provide flavor without all the sugar, making them a great choice for hydration throughout the day.

- **Creamy Coffee Drinks vs. Black Coffee or Coffee with Almond Milk:** Specialty coffee drinks like **lattes, frappuccinos**, and **mochas** can contain hundreds of calories from sugar, whipped cream, and syrups. Instead, opt for **black coffee** or **an Americano** with **a splash of unsweetened almond milk**. You can also add a dash of **cinnamon or nutmeg** for added flavor without the calories.

- **Alcoholic Cocktails vs. Simple Spirits**: Cocktails with sugary mixers, syrups, and cream can contain as many calories as a meal. Instead, choose a simple **spirit like vodka, gin**, or **tequila** mixed with **soda water** and a slice of **lime**. This reduces the calorie content significantly while still allowing you to enjoy a drink. **Light beer** or **dry wine** are also good choices, but it's essential to moderate your intake.

- **Milkshakes vs. Smoothies: Milkshakes** are often high in fat and sugar, making them a very calorie-dense treat. Swap milkshakes for **smoothies** made with **unsweetened almond milk, frozen fruit**, and **Greek yogurt**. This option provides the creamy texture you crave along with protein and fiber, making it a much more balanced and filling choice.

5.6.3 Enhancing Hydration with Flavor

Staying well-hydrated is essential for weight loss, as dehydration can sometimes be mistaken for hunger, leading to overeating. If you're not a fan of plain water, consider these smart ways to add flavor:

- **Fruit and Herb Infusions**: Make your water more enjoyable by adding fresh **fruits (like lemon, lime, berries)** and **herbs (like mint or basil)**. These simple infusions add flavor without adding calories.

- **Cold Herbal Teas**: Brew **herbal teas** like **peppermint, chamomile**, or **hibiscus**, and chill them in the refrigerator. These teas are naturally flavorful, contain no calories, and can be a great alternative to sugary drinks.

- **Sparkling Water with Citrus**: If you miss the fizziness of soda, **sparkling water** with a squeeze of **lemon, lime**, or **grapefruit** can be a great replacement. It satisfies the craving for something bubbly without the calories or sugar.

5.7 Making Swaps at Restaurants and Social Events: Eating Out without Overindulgence

5.7.1 Smart Swaps at Restaurants

When eating out, making small adjustments to your order can save hundreds of calories and help keep you on track with your goals without sacrificing flavor.

- **Appetizers and Starters**: Instead of calorie-heavy starters like **mozzarella sticks, wings,** or **fried calamari,** opt for lighter options like a **garden salad** (with dressing on the side), **shrimp cocktail,** or **broth-based soups** like **miso** or **minestrone**.

- **Main Courses**: Ask for **grilled or baked options** instead of fried, and choose a side of **steamed vegetables** or a **side salad** instead of **fries** or **creamed spinach**. For pasta dishes, request a **tomato-based sauce** instead of cream sauces.

- **Portion Control**: Restaurant portions are often much larger than what you'd serve yourself at home. Ask for **half of your meal to be boxed up** before it's brought to the table, or consider **sharing a main course** with someone else.

- **Desserts**: Desserts are often the biggest calorie traps. If you want to indulge, consider sharing a dessert with the table or opting for a lighter option like **fresh fruit** or **sorbet** instead of a heavy, cream-based dessert.

5.7.2 Navigating Social Events with Smart Swaps

Social events can be challenging because you're often not in control of the menu, and there's pressure to indulge. Here's how to make smart swaps while still enjoying yourself:

- **Potlucks**: If you're attending a **potluck**, bring a dish that aligns with your goals. For example, bring a **vegetable platter with hummus, grilled chicken skewers**, or a **quinoa salad**. This way, you're guaranteed to have at least one healthy option.

- **Buffets**: Buffets are notorious for encouraging overeating. Survey all the available options before filling your plate. Start with **salads and vegetables**, add a portion of **lean protein**, and keep **high-calorie sides** and **desserts** to a small portion.

- **Alcohol**: Social gatherings often involve alcohol. Choose **lighter options** like **white wine spritzers, light beer**, or **simple mixed drinks** (like vodka with soda water). Limit yourself to one or two drinks, and alternate with water to stay hydrated.

- **Dessert Table**: If there's a dessert table, allow yourself to enjoy a small taste rather than sampling everything. **Choose one or two treats** that you truly enjoy, and savor each bite.

5.8 Embracing Smart Swaps as a Lifestyle

5.8.1 Gradual Changes for Lasting Success

The key to making smart swaps a sustainable part of your life is to **implement them gradually**. Making too many changes at once can feel overwhelming, but starting with one or two easy swaps per meal can help you ease into a healthier routine. For example:

- **Start with Breakfast**: Focus on making your breakfast healthier—switch from sugary cereal to oats or swap cream in your coffee for almond milk.

- **Tackle Snacks**: Once you're comfortable with breakfast changes, move on to your snacks. Replace chips with veggies and hummus or swap candy bars for dark chocolate.

- **Transform Dinner**: Start experimenting with healthier cooking methods, like air frying or roasting, and introduce more vegetables into your evening meals.

Over time, these small changes will become habits, and you'll naturally find yourself choosing healthier options without feeling like you're missing out.

5.8.2 Finding Balance: Smart Swaps Without Sacrifice

The beauty of smart swaps is that they allow you to find **balance**. You're not giving up your favorite foods—you're just finding ways to make them work within your calorie and health goals. This mindset shift helps you avoid the feelings of deprivation that come with many diets and allows you to enjoy food in a healthy, sustainable way.

Instead of focusing on what you "can't" have, celebrate what you "can" have:

- **Enjoy burgers with lettuce wraps** instead of buns.

- **Indulge in ice cream** occasionally but make **banana nice cream** your go-to dessert.

- **Have your pasta** but mix it with **spiralized veggies** to lighten the load.

5.8.3 Learning to Listen to Your Body

Part of making smart swaps is also learning to listen to your body. Pay attention to how you feel after eating different foods. Do you feel energized, or do you feel sluggish? Do you feel satisfied or still hungry?

By tuning into your body's signals, you can make better decisions about the kinds of foods that make you feel your best. This might mean swapping out heavy meals that make you feel bloated for lighter, veggie-packed alternatives that leave you energized. Learning what your body needs and responding accordingly is key to creating a balanced, enjoyable, and sustainable approach to weight loss.

5.8.4 Celebrating the Journey

Finally, remember to celebrate your progress. Every small change is a victory, and every time you choose a smart swap over a less healthy option, you're taking a step towards better health. Weight loss is not about being perfect—it's about being consistent. The more you incorporate smart swaps, the more natural they will become, and the closer you will be to achieving your goals without feeling deprived.

5.8.5 Smart Swaps Summary: A Recap of Key Strategies

- **Breakfast**: Replace sugary cereals with oats, and swap buttered toast for avocado toast.

- **Lunch**: Choose whole-grain bread or wraps over white bread, and replace mayonnaise with mustard or Greek yogurt.

- **Dinner**: Grill or bake proteins instead of frying, swap white rice for cauliflower rice, and make vegetables the star of your plate.

- **Snacks and Desserts**: Opt for veggie chips over potato chips, dark chocolate over candy bars, and Greek yogurt over ice cream.

- **Drinks**: Swap sugary sodas for sparkling water, creamy lattes for black coffee, and calorie-heavy cocktails for simpler spirits.

Making these swaps part of your routine will help you stay on track, reduce unnecessary calorie intake, and enjoy your weight loss journey while still savoring delicious food.

Chapter 6: Building a Sustainable Mindset and Long-Term Habits

6.1 Why Mindset is the Key to Long-Term Success

6.1.1 The Role of Mental Attitude in Weight Loss

Weight loss is not just about eating less and exercising more—it's about creating a sustainable lifestyle that aligns with your goals and priorities. The journey often starts with the body, but it succeeds or fails based on the **mindset**. An individual's mental attitude influences their choices, motivation, and how they deal with setbacks. Understanding and nurturing a **growth mindset**—one where challenges are opportunities for learning—can make the difference between temporary weight loss and lifelong health.

- **Fixed vs. Growth Mindset**: A **fixed mindset** makes individuals believe that their abilities, qualities, or weight loss results are unchangeable. Statements like "I've always been overweight, and that's just who I am" are indicative of a fixed mindset. On the other hand, a **growth mindset** allows people to view challenges as opportunities and believe that change is always possible with effort and consistency. Adopting a growth mindset helps create the mental resilience needed for long-term weight loss success.

- **Changing the Focus from Outcomes to Habits**: Instead of focusing solely on the end result (such as losing 20 pounds), focus on the **daily habits** that will help you reach your goals. This mindset shift turns every day into an opportunity for small victories, reinforcing the idea that progress is made step by step.

6.1.2 The Impact of Emotional Triggers

Food is often more than sustenance—it is tied to emotions, comfort, and habit. Many people eat not because they're hungry but because they are sad, stressed, bored, or anxious. Understanding the role of **emotional eating** is crucial to overcoming it.

- **Identifying Triggers**: The first step in managing emotional eating is recognizing the specific triggers. These could be work stress, relationship issues, loneliness, boredom, or even specific events such as holidays. Keeping a **food and emotion journal** can help identify these triggers. By writing down what you eat, why you eat it, and how you feel before and after, patterns often become evident.

- **Breaking the Cycle**: Once triggers are identified, it's important to break the cycle by creating an **action plan**. For example, if stress at work is a trigger, instead of turning to food, consider going for a walk, practicing deep breathing exercises, or taking five minutes for meditation. By replacing emotional eating with a **positive action**, it becomes easier to cope with challenging feelings without turning to food.

6.1.3 The Power of Visualization and Goal Setting

Visualization and goal setting are powerful tools that can transform your approach to weight loss.

- **Visualizing Success: Visualization** is about imagining yourself reaching your goals. Visualizing yourself at your ideal weight, confidently wearing clothes you love, or feeling energized and healthy creates a positive mental image that motivates you. Spend a few minutes each day visualizing what success looks and feels like for you. This practice helps keep your long-term goals at the forefront of your mind.

- **Setting SMART Goals**: Weight loss goals should be **Specific, Measurable, Achievable, Relevant, and Time-bound (SMART)**. Instead of setting vague goals like "I want to lose weight," make them specific: "I will lose 10 pounds in three months by eating within my calorie budget and exercising four times a week." This approach gives you a clear target and a plan for how to achieve it.

6.1.4 Practicing Self-Compassion

Many people struggling with weight loss are overly critical of themselves, especially when they experience setbacks. Self-criticism, however, often leads to more emotional eating and a cycle of negativity. Practicing **self-compassion** is key to maintaining a healthy mindset during your journey.

- **Treating Yourself with Kindness**: Instead of being harsh when you make a mistake, imagine what you would say to a friend in the same situation. Offer yourself the same kindness. If you overeat at a social event, recognize that it's just one meal out of thousands and that it doesn't define your journey.

- **Affirmations and Positive Self-Talk**: Using **positive affirmations** can help reshape your internal dialogue. Repeating statements like "I am capable of making healthy choices," "I deserve to feel healthy and happy," or "Every step forward matters, no matter how small" can reinforce a positive mindset. This practice helps counteract negative self-talk and builds resilience.

6.2 Overcoming Common Challenges and Setbacks

6.2.1 Handling Plateaus

Weight loss plateaus are common and can be extremely frustrating. A plateau occurs when your body has adjusted to your new eating and exercise routine, and weight loss slows or stops. Here's how to navigate this challenging phase:

- **Understand Why Plateaus Happen**: During weight loss, your metabolism adjusts to your new weight and caloric intake. As you lose weight, your body requires fewer calories, which can lead to a plateau if you don't make changes. Understanding that plateaus are a natural part of the journey helps prevent discouragement.

- **Reassess Calorie Needs**: As your weight changes, so does your **Total Daily Energy Expenditure (TDEE)**. Recalculate your daily calorie needs and adjust your intake accordingly. Reducing your calorie intake by **100-200 calories** may be enough to overcome the plateau.

- **Change Up Your Exercise Routine**: Your body adapts to exercise over time, which means that the same workout becomes less effective. Introducing **high-**

intensity interval training (HIIT), trying new activities like **strength training, yoga**, or even just changing the intensity or duration of your workouts can jumpstart progress.

- **Focus on Non-Scale Victories (NSVs)**: Weight isn't the only measure of progress. Notice **other improvements** like increased energy, better sleep, looser clothes, or feeling stronger. These NSVs are important indicators that you're on the right track, even if the scale isn't moving.

6.2.2 Navigating Social Pressure and Expectations

Social situations can be one of the most challenging parts of losing weight. Friends and family, though well-intentioned, can unknowingly pressure you to overeat or make choices that don't align with your goals.

- **Communicate Your Goals**: It's helpful to communicate your goals to those around you. Let them know that you're working on your health and appreciate their support. This doesn't mean you need to share every detail, but simply making your intentions clear can reduce social pressure.

- **Setting Boundaries**: There may be times when friends or family push food on you or question your choices. Practice **assertive but polite responses**. For example, "Thank you, but I'm full," or "That looks delicious, but I'm trying to stick to my plan right now." Setting boundaries isn't about being rude—it's about honoring your own needs.

- **Dealing with Food Pushers**: Some people, known as **food pushers**, will persist even after you've said no. This can be particularly common in cultural or family settings where food is an expression of love. In these cases, you can take small portions, compliment the cook, and emphasize your appreciation without overindulging.

6.2.3 Overcoming Binge Eating Tendencies

Binge eating is a common challenge, especially for those who have followed restrictive diets in the past. It's characterized by eating large quantities of food in a short period, often accompanied by feelings of guilt or loss of control. Here are strategies to break the binge-restrict cycle:

- **Avoid Restriction**: One of the biggest causes of binge eating is **over-restriction**. When people deprive themselves of certain foods, they eventually crave them intensely, leading to a binge. Incorporate **moderate amounts** of all foods you enjoy into your diet to avoid feeling deprived. Knowing that no food is completely off-limits helps reduce the urgency to overeat.

- **Practice Mindful Eating: Mindful eating** involves paying attention to your food, eating slowly, and savoring every bite. This practice helps you recognize your body's hunger and fullness cues, reducing the likelihood of overeating. When you eat mindfully, you're more in tune with what you're eating and why.

- **Seek Professional Help**: If binge eating is a frequent issue that's affecting your health and well-being, consider seeking help from a **therapist or dietitian** specializing in **eating disorders**. Professional support can provide tools and strategies tailored to your specific needs.

6.2.4 Dealing with Cravings

Cravings are natural, but giving in to every craving can make it difficult to stay on track. Here are strategies for managing and reducing cravings:

- **Identify True Hunger vs. Emotional Hunger**: Ask yourself whether you're truly hungry or if you're craving something for emotional reasons. True hunger often comes on gradually, whereas emotional hunger is sudden and tied to specific cravings (like sweets or salty snacks). Understanding the difference can help you decide whether to eat or find another activity to cope.

- **Distract Yourself**: Cravings often pass if you give them some time. Try distracting yourself with an activity that keeps your hands and mind busy—go for a walk, read a book, or engage in a hobby you enjoy. If the craving subsides, you know it wasn't true hunger.

- **Healthy Swaps for Common Cravings**: If you do decide to indulge a craving, try to make it a healthier version. For example, if you're craving ice cream, try **Greek yogurt with berries**. If you're craving salty snacks, opt for **air-popped popcorn** instead of chips. Finding **lower-calorie alternatives** helps satisfy the craving without derailing your progress.

- **Allow for Moderation**: Allowing yourself to have a small portion of something you're craving can help reduce the desire to overeat. For example, having one square of dark chocolate can be more satisfying than trying to ignore the craving entirely, which could lead to a binge later on.

6.3 Building Consistent Habits: The Foundation of Long-Term Success

6.3.1 The Importance of Habit Formation

Creating lasting habits is essential for maintaining weight loss long term. It's the daily choices that ultimately define success. Understanding how habits are formed and leveraging that knowledge to build healthy routines can transform the weight loss journey from a temporary challenge into a permanent lifestyle.

- **The Habit Loop**: Habits are made up of a **cue, routine, and reward**—known as the **habit loop**. For example, if your cue is **feeling stressed**, your routine might be **eating a snack**, and the reward is the **temporary comfort** the food provides. To change a habit, you can keep the cue and reward but replace the routine. Instead of eating a snack when stressed, try replacing it with **a brisk walk or deep breathing**.

- **Start Small**: One of the biggest mistakes people make is trying to change too much at once. Instead, focus on **one habit at a time**. For example, if you want to start exercising, start by walking for **10 minutes a day**. Once that becomes consistent, gradually increase the time or intensity. Small, consistent steps are much more effective in the long term.

- **Anchor Habits: Anchor habits** are behaviors you tie to existing habits to help establish new routines. For instance, if you already brush your teeth every morning, you could anchor a new habit to it, like **doing five minutes of stretching** right afterward. Tying new habits to established routines helps integrate them into your daily life without feeling overwhelming.

6.3.2 Establishing a Routine that Supports Your Goals

Building a daily routine that aligns with your weight loss goals creates consistency and reduces the need for willpower. Here are some tips for building routines around nutrition, exercise, and self-care:

- **Meal Planning and Preparation**: Taking time each week to plan and prepare meals helps ensure that you have healthy options available, making it easier to stick to your calorie goals. **Meal prepping** can include cooking a big batch of grains, roasting vegetables, and grilling proteins that you can mix and match throughout the week.

- **Setting Regular Mealtimes**: Establishing consistent meal times can help regulate hunger and prevent overeating. Eating at similar times each day keeps your body's hunger cues in check, reducing the risk of mindless snacking. If you find yourself getting too hungry between meals, plan for a **healthy snack** like an apple with almond butter.

- **Exercise as a Non-Negotiable**: Consistent physical activity is an important habit for weight loss and overall health. Find an activity you enjoy, whether it's **dancing, swimming, hiking,** or **strength training,** and build it into your schedule. Treat your workout like any other important appointment—make it non-negotiable.

6.3.3 Mindful Eating as a Habit

Mindful eating involves being fully present during meals, paying attention to hunger and fullness cues, and savoring each bite. Developing a mindful eating habit helps prevent overeating and creates a more enjoyable eating experience.

- **Eliminate Distractions**: Eating in front of the TV or while scrolling through your phone makes it easy to consume more food than you intended. When eating, try to eliminate distractions and focus solely on your meal.

- **Slow Down**: It takes about **20 minutes** for the brain to register that you're full. Eating slowly allows your body time to catch up, reducing the likelihood of overeating. Practice setting down your utensils between bites and chewing thoroughly.

- **Check-In with Hunger and Fullness Levels**: Before eating, rate your hunger on a scale from **1-10**, with 1 being extremely hungry and 10 being overly full. Ideally, you want to start eating when you're around a **3 or 4** and stop when you're around a **7**—comfortably satisfied, but not stuffed.

6.3.4 Building an Environment that Supports Success

Your environment plays a significant role in shaping your habits and making it easier or harder to achieve your goals. Creating a **supportive environment** makes it more likely that you'll succeed without having to rely solely on willpower.

- **Stock Up on Healthy Foods**: Keep your kitchen stocked with healthy options like **fresh fruits, vegetables, lean proteins, whole grains**, and **healthy snacks**. When nutritious foods are easily accessible, you're more likely to make healthier choices.

- **Remove Temptations**: Remove foods from your home that you tend to overeat. If you struggle with overeating certain snacks, don't keep them in your kitchen. Instead, make them a treat you enjoy only occasionally and deliberately, perhaps when dining out or during special occasions.

- **Keep Exercise Gear Handy**: If exercise is part of your weight loss goal, make it easy to be active. Keep your **exercise clothes, sneakers**, and **equipment** in a place that's convenient. If you're more likely to work out in the morning, set your workout clothes out the night before.

6.3.5 Building Accountability into Your Habits

Accountability can significantly increase your chances of success. Knowing that someone else is aware of your goals can provide motivation and support.

- **Accountability Partners**: Find a friend, family member, or colleague with similar health goals, and become accountability partners. You can check in with each other regularly, celebrate successes, and provide support during challenges.

- **Journaling**: Keeping a **food journal** can help you stay accountable to yourself. Record what you eat, your workouts, and how you feel each day. Reflecting on your progress and recognizing your wins can boost your motivation.

- **Join a Community**: Online communities or local support groups focused on health and wellness can provide valuable support. Sharing your journey with others and seeing their successes and challenges can be motivating and make you feel less alone.

6.4 Building Resilience and Staying Motivated

6.4.1 Understanding Motivation and Discipline

Motivation can be fleeting—it's often high at the beginning of a weight loss journey but may wane over time. Relying solely on motivation can be problematic. This is where **discipline** and habit formation come into play.

- **Intrinsic vs. Extrinsic Motivation**: Motivation can be **intrinsic** (coming from within) or **extrinsic** (influenced by external factors). **Intrinsic motivation,** such as wanting to feel more energized or healthier, tends to be more sustainable. **Extrinsic motivation,** like wanting to fit into a particular outfit or impress others, can help get you started but may not last as long. Connecting your goals to a deeper, intrinsic "why" helps maintain focus even when motivation wanes.

- **Relying on Habits, Not Motivation**: Discipline and well-formed habits can carry you through times when motivation is low. Instead of waiting to feel motivated to exercise, build it into your daily routine until it becomes automatic—just like brushing your teeth.

6.4.2 Celebrating Wins, No Matter How Small

Celebrating milestones along the way helps maintain a positive attitude and keeps you motivated. Recognizing progress beyond just the number on the scale reinforces that health and weight loss are about much more than aesthetics.

- **Non-Scale Victories (NSVs)**: Focus on the many non-scale victories that come with weight loss and healthy living. These could be **fitting into old clothes, having more energy, improving your sleep quality,** or **noticing increased strength during workouts**. Celebrating these wins helps keep you motivated, especially during times when the scale isn't moving.

- **Reward Yourself**: Reward yourself in ways that support your goals. Instead of using food as a reward, consider treating yourself to a **spa day, new workout clothes, a book you've wanted**, or any other non-food reward that feels good to you.

6.4.3 Developing a Growth Mindset Around Setbacks

Setbacks are a natural part of any journey, and how you respond to them determines your long-term success.

- **View Setbacks as Learning Opportunities**: Instead of seeing setbacks as failures, view them as **learning opportunities**. If you overeat, reflect on what led to it—were you overly hungry because you skipped a meal? Were you stressed or tired? Use these reflections to develop strategies for the future.

- **Practice Resilience**: Resilience is the ability to bounce back after a setback. If you have an off day, remind yourself that one day doesn't define your progress. The key is to keep moving forward without letting one misstep turn into a week or month of giving up.

6.4.4 Staying Connected to Your "Why"

Staying connected to your deeper reasons for wanting to lose weight is crucial for staying motivated, especially during difficult times.

- **Create a Vision Board**: A **vision board** is a visual representation of your goals. It can include pictures, quotes, and other images that remind you why you started. Keep your vision board somewhere you'll see it daily to help you stay focused on your end goal.

- **Write a Letter to Yourself**: Write a letter to your future self, describing why you want to lose weight, how you want to feel, and what reaching your goal will mean to you. Reading this letter when you're feeling unmotivated can help reignite your commitment to your goals.

6.5 Finding Joy in the Journey

6.5.1 Redefining Your Relationship with Food

For many people, weight loss can feel like a constant battle with food—counting calories, avoiding favorite treats, and feeling guilty after eating certain things. Finding **joy in the journey** is about redefining your relationship with food and focusing on **nourishment and enjoyment.**

- **Enjoy All Foods in Moderation**: Food isn't inherently good or bad—it's all about balance. Learning to enjoy **all foods in moderation** allows you to indulge in your favorites without guilt. If you're craving a slice of cake, have it—but savor it, eat it mindfully, and remember that one slice isn't going to make or break your progress.

- **Focus on Nourishing Your Body**: Shift the focus from restriction to **nourishment.** Instead of thinking about what you need to cut out, think about what you can add to your diet that will make you feel good. Adding **colorful vegetables, lean proteins, healthy fats**, and **whole grains** to your meals helps nourish your body and keeps you satisfied.

6.5.2 Finding Joy in Movement

Exercise shouldn't be a punishment for what you ate—it should be a way to celebrate what your body can do. Finding an activity you genuinely enjoy makes it easier to stay consistent with exercise.

- **Try Different Activities**: There's no one-size-fits-all when it comes to exercise. Experiment with different activities until you find what you enjoy. Whether it's **dancing, yoga, weightlifting, swimming, or hiking,** finding something you love makes it easier to stay active consistently.

- **Exercise with Friends**: Exercising with friends can make it more enjoyable and help you stay motivated. Join a **class**, go for **group hikes**, or try a **fitness challenge** together. Making exercise a social activity creates a positive association with it and helps make it a lasting habit.

- **Celebrate What Your Body Can Do**: Instead of focusing on how your body looks, celebrate what it can do. Notice your **strength**, your **endurance**, and the **progress** you make over time. Whether it's lifting heavier weights, running further, or holding a yoga pose longer, celebrating your physical capabilities is a great way to stay motivated.

6.5.3 Making Self-Care a Priority

Self-care is an important but often overlooked part of the weight loss journey. Taking care of your mental, emotional, and physical well-being creates a positive environment for sustainable weight loss.

- **Prioritize Rest and Recovery**: Rest is just as important as exercise. Make sure you're getting enough **quality sleep** each night, as lack of sleep can lead to increased hunger and cravings. Listen to your body and take **rest days** when needed to allow for recovery.

- **Stress Management**: Chronic stress can lead to emotional eating and weight gain. Incorporate **stress-reducing activities** into your daily routine, such as **meditation, journaling, yoga**, or **deep breathing exercises**. Managing stress helps prevent overeating and keeps your mental health in check.

- **Practice Gratitude**: Taking a few moments each day to reflect on what you're grateful for can help improve your overall mindset and make the journey more enjoyable. Gratitude shifts the focus away from what's lacking to what's already good, fostering a positive attitude toward your body and progress.

6.6 Integrating Long-Term Habits for a Sustainable Lifestyle

6.6.1 Designing a Maintenance Plan

Once you reach your weight loss goal, the journey isn't over. The focus shifts to **maintaining your progress** and integrating the habits that got you there into your permanent lifestyle.

- **Transitioning from Deficit to Maintenance**: The biggest difference between weight loss and maintenance is calorie intake. Slowly increase your daily calorie intake to reach **maintenance calories**— the amount of energy your body needs to maintain its current weight. This transition should be done gradually, monitoring your weight and adjusting as needed to avoid regaining lost weight.

- **Stay Active**: Exercise remains important for maintenance. The goal isn't to burn calories but to support your health, boost your mood, and keep your body strong. Find activities you enjoy and aim for a mix of **cardiovascular, strength training**, and **flexibility exercises** to keep your body balanced.

- **Continue Meal Planning and Prepping**: Planning and preparing meals helps maintain your weight long-term. By having healthy options available, you're less likely to make impulsive, less nutritious choices. The structure that helped you lose weight will also help you keep it off.

6.6.2 The Power of Routine and Flexibility

Routine provides structure, but flexibility is what makes a healthy lifestyle sustainable.

- **Balancing Routine with Flexibility**: Routine helps keep healthy habits consistent, but being overly rigid can lead to burnout. For example, if you're used to exercising every morning but one day you're tired or have an early appointment, don't see it as a failure if you miss your workout. Instead, adapt and plan a different activity later in the day or the following day.

- **Learning to Trust Your Body**: Long-term success is about trusting your body's cues and learning to eat intuitively. As you become more comfortable with your new habits, you'll find that your body naturally craves **nutritious foods** and enjoys movement. Allow yourself flexibility while still maintaining the principles that have supported your success.

6.6.3 Lifelong Learning and Adaptation

Your needs and circumstances will change over time. Staying healthy means being open to **learning and adapting** as life evolves.

- **Keep Educating Yourself**: The more you understand about **nutrition, fitness**, and **mental health**, the better equipped you'll be to make informed decisions. Stay curious—read books, listen to podcasts, or take courses that support your health goals.

- **Adapt to Life Changes**: Major life events—like moving, starting a new job, having children, or aging—will change your lifestyle and routines. The key is to adapt your habits to fit your new circumstances. If you're pressed for time, focus on shorter, more intense workouts. If you're feeling more stressed, incorporate more **relaxation practices**. Flexibility and adaptability are the cornerstones of long-term success.

6.6.4 Conclusion: Building a Lifestyle of Balance

Building a sustainable mindset and long-term habits is about creating a lifestyle that is **balanced and enjoyable**. Weight loss doesn't have to mean deprivation, and health isn't about perfection. It's about making choices each day that align with your goals while still allowing room for **enjoyment, flexibility**, and **self-compassion**.

By focusing on mindset, overcoming challenges, building consistent habits, staying resilient, and finding joy in the journey, you create a foundation for lifelong health. The key is to keep going, one step at a time, and remember that every small choice contributes to your overall well-being. Celebrate your progress, learn from setbacks, and stay connected to your goals—because this journey is not just about losing weight; it's about gaining a healthier, happier, and more fulfilled version of yourself.

Chapter 7: The Social Dynamics of Weight Loss

7.1 Understanding Social Influences on Weight Loss

7.1.1 How Social Relationships Affect Eating Habits

Our eating habits are not formed in a vacuum—they are shaped largely by our **social environment**. The people around us influence what we eat, how much we eat, and even our attitudes towards exercise. Understanding the impact of social relationships on eating behavior can provide insights into how to navigate social situations without jeopardizing weight loss goals.

- **Family Dynamics**: Families often play a significant role in shaping eating habits, especially during childhood. **Family traditions**, **meal patterns**, and **food preferences** established at a young age can influence eating behaviors well into adulthood. For example, if you grew up in a household where high-calorie, comfort foods were used to celebrate every occasion, you might struggle to break free from these habits.

- **Friends and Peers**: Friends and peers have a powerful influence on eating habits and physical activity levels. **Social gatherings** often revolve around food, and the people we spend time with can either encourage healthy habits or lead us toward overeating and sedentary behavior. Studies have shown that people are more likely to adopt the eating habits of those they spend time with, meaning that if your friends frequently dine out or eat unhealthy foods, you may be more likely to do the same.

- **Social Comparison: Social comparison** plays a significant role in shaping attitudes toward weight loss. People often compare themselves to friends, colleagues, or even strangers on social media, which can either motivate or discourage them. If your social circle places a high value on health and fitness, you may feel encouraged to pursue similar goals. Conversely, comparing yourself to those with unattainable or unrealistic standards can lead to feelings of inadequacy and disheartenment.

7.1.2 The Impact of Culture on Weight Loss

Cultural influences play a crucial role in shaping our relationship with food, body image, and weight loss. Different cultures have unique attitudes toward food, and these attitudes can either support or hinder weight loss efforts.

- **Cultural Celebrations and Food**: Many cultures use food as a central part of celebrations, festivals, and rituals. Whether it's family gatherings, holidays, or religious events, food is often an essential part of the experience. This cultural emphasis on food can make it challenging for individuals who are trying to lose weight, as they may feel pressured to eat traditional dishes that are high in calories.

- **Body Image and Cultural Expectations**: Different cultures have varying ideals of beauty and body image. In some cultures, a fuller figure is associated with health, wealth, and attractiveness, while in others, thinness is idealized. These cultural expectations can create conflicting feelings about weight loss. Some individuals may face resistance from their communities if they start losing weight and no longer fit the cultural norm.

- **Adapting Traditional Foods**: One way to balance cultural expectations and weight loss goals is to adapt traditional foods to make them healthier. For example, if a traditional dish is typically deep-fried, consider baking or air-frying instead. By finding ways to modify traditional dishes while preserving their cultural significance, individuals can enjoy their heritage without compromising their health.

7.1.3 Social Media and Its Influence on Weight Loss

Social media is a powerful tool that shapes our attitudes, behaviors, and perceptions about weight loss and fitness. It can provide support, motivation, and information, but it can also create unrealistic expectations and pressure.

- **The Positive Side of Social Media: Social media** can provide a sense of community and support for those looking to lose weight. **Fitness influencers, health coaches**, and **weight loss groups** on platforms like Instagram, TikTok, and Facebook can be sources of motivation and accountability. These platforms allow users to share their progress, celebrate victories, and connect with others on a similar journey.

- **The Negative Side of Social Media**: On the flip side, social media can create **unrealistic expectations** through heavily edited images, filters, and "highlight reels" that portray an idealized version of weight loss. The constant exposure to seemingly perfect bodies and extreme fitness routines can lead to **body dissatisfaction** and **feelings of inadequacy**. It's crucial to remember that many of the images shared on social media are not reflective of reality, and comparing yourself to these images can be detrimental to mental health.

- **Curate Your Feed**: To create a supportive social media environment, **curate your feed** to include positive, realistic, and uplifting content. Follow accounts that promote **body positivity, healthy habits**, and **balanced approaches** to weight loss.

Unfollow accounts that make you feel bad about yourself or promote extreme or unhealthy practices.

7.1.4 Understanding Group Dynamics and Weight Loss

Group dynamics can play an essential role in weight loss. Being part of a group—whether it's family, friends, coworkers, or an online community—can significantly influence your progress.

- **Positive Peer Pressure: Positive peer pressure** can be a powerful motivator for weight loss. For example, if your friends enjoy working out, you're more likely to join them and stay consistent. Group activities such as **group fitness classes, hiking,** or **walking clubs** can provide both accountability and enjoyment, making it easier to stick to a healthy routine.

- **Negative Peer Pressure:** Conversely, **negative peer pressure** can lead to setbacks. Friends or family members who don't share your health goals may encourage you to skip workouts, indulge in unhealthy foods, or criticize your efforts. Learning how to manage this pressure is crucial for maintaining long-term habits.

7.2 Building a Supportive Social Environment

7.2.1 The Role of Social Support in Weight Loss

Social support is one of the most significant factors that influence success in weight loss. Whether it's support from family, friends, coworkers, or online communities, having a network that encourages and uplifts you can make all the difference.

- **Emotional Support: Emotional support** involves having people who listen to you, empathize with your challenges, and celebrate your successes. Emotional support can come from friends, family members, or support groups. It helps to have someone to talk to when you're struggling with motivation or facing setbacks.

- **Practical Support: Practical support** includes tangible assistance, such as helping with meal prep, cooking healthy dishes together, or babysitting so you can go to the gym. Having someone who shares practical responsibilities can make weight loss efforts more manageable.

- **Accountability Partners:** An **accountability partner** can be a friend or family member who is also working on their health or is supportive of your journey. They can help you stay on track by checking in regularly, exercising together, or simply providing encouragement. Knowing that someone else is aware of your goals and progress can help keep you motivated and committed.

7.2.2 Creating a Weight Loss-Friendly Home Environment

The environment you live in plays a significant role in your success with weight loss. Creating a home environment that supports your health goals makes it easier to stay on track and reduces the need for willpower.

- **Kitchen Organization**: Keep your kitchen organized and stocked with **healthy options**. Make healthy foods like **fruits, vegetables, lean proteins, whole grains**, and **nuts** easily accessible, while keeping less healthy options out of sight. For example, place fruits and vegetables at eye level in the fridge and store snacks in opaque containers.

- **Involving Family Members**: If you live with family members, involve them in your weight loss journey. Explain your goals and ask for their support. Encourage **healthy family meals** that everyone can enjoy, rather than preparing separate dishes for yourself. Getting the whole family involved can create a positive environment where everyone benefits from healthier choices.

- **Creating Exercise-Friendly Spaces**: Make exercise a part of your home environment by creating a space where you can work out comfortably. Whether it's a corner of your living room, a spare room, or a section of your garage, having a dedicated space with **exercise equipment** like dumbbells, resistance bands, or a yoga mat can make it easier to stay consistent.

7.2.3 Building Healthy Relationships Around Food

The relationships we have with others often revolve around food—whether it's family dinners, gatherings with friends, or celebrations. Learning to build healthy relationships around food involves finding ways to enjoy these experiences without compromising your weight loss goals.

- **Reframing Food-Centric Social Events**: Instead of letting social events revolve solely around food, find other activities to enjoy together. For example, if you're planning a gathering with friends, consider activities like **hiking, a fitness class**, or **a game night** instead of just a meal. This helps shift the focus away from food and makes socializing less about eating.

- **Setting Boundaries with Loved Ones**: It can be challenging when family members or friends are not supportive of your weight loss efforts or don't understand why you're making changes. Setting boundaries is important. For instance, if you have a family member who insists on offering you second servings, politely but firmly decline by saying, "I appreciate it, but I'm full." Setting boundaries helps protect your health goals without damaging relationships.

- **Navigating Family Meals**: Family meals can be challenging, especially if traditional dishes are high in calories. Consider contributing a **healthier dish** to share or adapting recipes to be lighter. This allows you to stay on track while still enjoying the communal experience.

7.3 Strategies for Managing Social Pressures

7.3.1 Navigating Social Events and Parties

Social events, such as parties, gatherings, and celebrations, can be challenging for those trying to lose weight due to the abundance of high-calorie foods and the pressure to indulge. Here are strategies to navigate these situations without feeling deprived:

- **Eat Before You Go**: If you know that the food at a social event will not align with your weight loss goals, **eat a healthy meal or snack** before you go. This will help reduce your hunger, making it easier to say no to less healthy options. Eating something high in **protein and fiber**—such as **Greek yogurt with berries** or **a salad with grilled chicken**—can keep you full and satisfied.

- **Scan the Buffet Before Filling Your Plate**: When at a buffet, take a moment to **scan all the options** before deciding what to put on your plate. This helps you choose what you genuinely want and avoid overeating. Aim to fill your plate mostly with **vegetables, lean proteins,** and **a small portion of your favorite indulgence**.

- **Portion Control and Mindful Indulgence**: If you want to indulge in some of the high-calorie foods available, do so mindfully. Take small portions, savor every bite, and stop when you're satisfied. By allowing yourself to enjoy these foods in moderation, you reduce the likelihood of overindulging later.

7.3.2 Responding to Food Pushers

Food pushers are people who try to persuade you to eat more or eat foods you're trying to avoid, often out of love, tradition, or social expectations. Here are some ways to handle food pushers without causing offense:

- **Polite Decline**: Politely but firmly decline their offer. For example, you could say, "Thank you, it looks delicious, but I'm not hungry right now." Being polite but direct is often enough for most people to understand and respect your decision.

- **Divert the Conversation**: Sometimes food pushers are persistent, especially if they don't understand your reasons for refusing. **Diverting the conversation** away from food can help shift the focus. Ask about their day, bring up a new topic, or compliment something about the event. This distraction can help steer them away from focusing on what you are or aren't eating.

- **Take Control**: In situations where it's difficult to avoid pressure, such as family gatherings, **taking control of what's being served** can be helpful. Offer to bring a dish or help with the cooking. This allows you to prepare something you know is aligned with your goals while still contributing to the meal.

7.3.3 Dealing with Social Comparison

Social comparison can be a significant source of discouragement during a weight loss journey. Whether it's comparing yourself to friends, colleagues, or influencers on social media, these comparisons can undermine your progress. Here are ways to manage social comparison:

- **Focus on Your Own Journey**: Remember that everyone's journey is different. Each person's body, metabolism, lifestyle, and challenges are unique. Comparing your progress to someone else's doesn't account for all these differences. Focus on your own **goals, progress**, and **small victories**, and celebrate what you've achieved, no matter how small.

- **Unfollow Triggers on Social Media**: If certain accounts on social media make you feel less confident or discourage you, consider **unfollowing them**. Instead, follow accounts that promote **body positivity, realistic progress**, and **healthy lifestyles**. Creating a supportive social media environment can help you stay positive and motivated.

- **Turn Comparison into Inspiration**: If you do find yourself comparing yourself to someone else, try to **reframe** it as inspiration. Look at what that person is doing and ask yourself what you can learn from them. Maybe they are consistent with their exercise or have a balanced approach to eating—identify what aspects inspire you and incorporate them into your journey.

7.4 The Importance of Community in Weight Loss

7.4.1 Finding a Supportive Community

A supportive community can provide motivation, accountability, and encouragement throughout your weight loss journey. Whether it's an in-person group or an online community, having people who understand and share your goals can make all the difference.

- **Join a Weight Loss Group: Weight loss groups** like **Weight Watchers, Overeaters Anonymous**, or local **fitness challenges** can provide a structured environment with regular meetings, check-ins, and support. Being part of a group helps create a sense of accountability and community, making it easier to stay committed.

- **Online Communities**: Online communities, forums, and social media groups offer a sense of connection and support for those who may not have access to in-person groups. Platforms like **Reddit, Facebook**, or even **dedicated apps** have groups where members share their challenges, victories, and tips. Being part of an online community allows you to find others with similar experiences and exchange support.

- **Fitness Classes and Groups**: Participating in **fitness classes**—whether in-person or online—creates an environment of encouragement and camaraderie. Classes like **spin, yoga, dance**, or **martial arts** can provide a motivating group atmosphere. Group activities tend to encourage consistency and a sense of accountability, which are crucial for long-term success.

7.4.2 Sharing Your Goals with Your Community

Sharing your weight loss goals with others can help you stay committed and motivated. When you share your goals, you're not only holding yourself accountable, but you're also inviting others to support and encourage you.

- **Share with Friends and Family**: Tell close friends and family about your goals and ask for their support. Let them know how they can help, whether it's through **words of encouragement, joining you for a walk**, or simply **respecting your food choices**. Sharing your goals creates a sense of accountability, and having others aware of your journey can provide much-needed motivation.

- **Document Your Journey**: Consider documenting your journey publicly or privately. You could start a **blog, a social media account**, or even a **private journal**. Sharing your progress, challenges, and reflections can create a sense of accountability. It also allows you to track your growth and look back on how far you've come.

- **Celebrate Together**: When you achieve a milestone, share it with your community. Celebrating milestones together—whether it's **losing 10 pounds, completing a fitness challenge**, or simply **feeling healthier—**

creates a sense of accomplishment and reinforces the idea that weight loss is a shared journey.

7.4.3 Finding Like-Minded People

Finding people with similar goals and values can help you stay consistent and motivated. These individuals understand the challenges you're facing and can provide support when you need it most.

- **Join Fitness or Cooking Clubs**: Clubs centered around **fitness, healthy cooking,** or **wellness** can provide opportunities to meet like-minded people. Whether it's a local **running club, a hiking group**, or a **healthy cooking class**, these activities allow you to meet others with similar interests and goals.

- **Network Through Friends**: Let your friends know about your goals and interests. They may be able to connect you with others who share similar goals. Meeting friends of friends who are also interested in weight loss or healthy living can help expand your supportive network.

- **Online Networking**: Use online platforms to network with others who share your interests. For example, if you enjoy cooking, join **Facebook groups** dedicated to healthy recipes. If you enjoy yoga, participate in **online yoga challenges**. These platforms allow you to connect with others regardless of location.

7.5 Leveraging Social Accountability for Motivation

7.5.1 Understanding the Power of Accountability

Accountability can be one of the most powerful tools for motivation in weight loss. Knowing that someone else is aware of your goals and progress can provide extra motivation to stay consistent, even when you don't feel like it.

- **Types of Accountability**: Accountability can come from **partners, groups**, or **personal tracking**. **Partners** are individuals who directly check in with you and support you. **Groups** provide a broader sense of accountability, and **personal tracking**—such as keeping a journal or using an app—holds you accountable to yourself. Using a combination of these can provide the most effective results.

- **Accountability Partners**: An **accountability partner** could be a friend, family member, coworker, or even someone you meet through an online community. Ideally, your partner is someone who understands your goals and is supportive of your efforts. Regular check-ins—whether daily, weekly, or monthly—allow you to share your progress, celebrate successes, and discuss challenges.

7.5.2 Group Challenges and Fitness Competitions

Participating in group challenges and competitions can add an element of fun and motivation to your weight loss journey.

- **Fitness Challenges**: Participating in a **30-day fitness challenge**, a **step-count challenge**, or a **push-up challenge** with friends or coworkers adds a sense of friendly competition and motivation. These challenges encourage consistency, especially when you know others are doing it with you. Fitness apps, social media groups, and local gyms often host group challenges that you can join.

- **Weight Loss Competitions**: Some people are motivated by **weight loss competitions**, where participants compete to see who can lose the most weight over a set period. These competitions can provide motivation but should be approached with caution. The focus should always be on healthy weight loss, not extreme or unsustainable methods. Set reasonable and healthy goals, and avoid any pressure to lose weight too quickly.

- **Team-Based Activities**: Activities that require teamwork—such as **relay races, team sports**, or even **charity walks**—provide accountability and build a sense of camaraderie. Working toward a collective goal adds motivation and helps create a bond with others, making the experience more enjoyable.

7.5.3 Apps and Technology for Social Accountability

Technology has made it easier than ever to stay accountable and motivated through social connections. Using apps and online platforms to track progress, connect with others, and celebrate successes can help keep you on track.

- **Fitness Tracking Apps**: Apps like **MyFitnessPal, Fitbit**, and **Noom** allow you to track your food intake, physical activity, and progress. Many of these apps have social features, allowing you to connect with friends, join groups, and share your progress. Seeing others' progress can be motivating, and sharing your own adds a layer of accountability.

- **Social Fitness Platforms**: Platforms like **Strava** allow you to track your workouts and share them with your network. You can see your friends' activities, give them "kudos," and join group challenges. These social fitness platforms create a sense of community and competition that keeps you motivated.

- **Digital Accountability Groups**: Online programs and apps like **DietBet** or **HealthyWage** allow users to participate in weight loss challenges, with the added motivation of financial incentives. Participants bet on themselves to lose weight, and those who achieve their goals win a portion of the pot. This adds both social accountability and a financial incentive to stay on track.

7.6 Finding Balance in Social Settings

7.6.1 Balancing Social Life with Weight Loss Goals

Balancing a social life with weight loss goals can be challenging, especially when social events often involve food and drinks. Finding ways to enjoy social gatherings while staying on track with your goals is key to creating a sustainable lifestyle.

- **Being Selective**: Not every social event requires you to indulge. Be **selective** about which events are worth making exceptions for. For example, you might choose to indulge at your best friend's wedding but decide to stay on track at a casual Friday night gathering. By being selective, you can still enjoy special occasions without derailing your progress.

- **Alternatives to Drinking Alcohol**: Alcohol can be a significant source of empty calories, and social pressure to drink can be strong. If you want to reduce alcohol consumption, try **mocktails, sparkling water with lime**, or **soda water** with a splash of fruit juice. These alternatives allow you to still have a drink in hand without the excess calories.

- **Focus on the Social Aspect**: Instead of focusing on the food or drinks at social events, shift your focus to the social experience. **Engage in conversations, dance**, or **play games**—these activities help keep your mind off food and make the event more enjoyable without overindulgence.

7.6.2 Eating Out at Restaurants with Friends and Family

Dining out at restaurants is a common social activity, but it can be challenging when you're trying to lose weight. With a few strategies, you can enjoy dining out without compromising your goals.

- **Review the Menu in Advance**: Many restaurants post their menus online. Reviewing the menu ahead of time allows you to make an informed decision about what to order. Look for dishes that are **grilled, baked, steamed**, or **roasted**, and opt for **vegetables or salads** as sides.

- **Customizing Your Order**: Don't be afraid to **customize your order**. Ask for sauces on the side, substitute fries for a salad, or request grilled instead of fried. Most restaurants are happy to accommodate special requests, and these small changes can significantly reduce the calorie content of your meal.

- **Be Mindful of Portions**: Restaurant portions are often much larger than what you would serve at home. Consider **sharing a dish** with a friend or asking for a **to-go box** when your meal arrives and putting half of it away for later. This helps with portion control and prevents overeating.

7.6.3 Maintaining Social Relationships During Weight Loss

Weight loss can change the dynamics of social relationships, especially when friends and family may not share your goals. Maintaining healthy social relationships while staying true to your goals is crucial for long-term success.

- **Communicate Openly**: Open communication is key when it comes to maintaining relationships during weight loss. Let your friends and family know what you're working toward and why it's important to you. This helps them understand your perspective and can reduce misunderstandings or negative feelings.

- **Be Patient with Loved Ones**: Not everyone will understand your goals, and some people may even be resistant to your changes. **Be patient** with loved ones who may need time to adjust. Remember that your decision to lose weight is about your health and well-being, and it may take others time to understand your new habits.

- **Lead by Example**: Your journey may inspire others. As you continue to make positive changes, those around you may become interested in adopting similar habits. Instead of pushing others to change, lead by example—invite friends for **walks**, share **healthy recipes**, or introduce them to **fun activities**. Leading by example allows others to see the benefits of a healthy lifestyle without feeling pressured.

7.7 Conclusion: Leveraging Social Dynamics for Long-Term Success

Weight loss is a deeply personal journey, but it's also one that is heavily influenced by social dynamics. The people you surround yourself with, the social situations you find yourself in, and the cultural and societal pressures you face all impact your ability to lose weight and maintain it long-term.

This chapter has explored how to navigate social pressures, build a supportive environment, leverage community accountability, and find balance in social settings—all of which are essential for creating a sustainable, enjoyable, and successful weight loss journey.

The key takeaway is that you don't have to do it alone. **Surround yourself with people who uplift you, communicate your goals, and seek out communities** that share your values. By leveraging social dynamics positively, you can build a support network that helps you stay motivated, overcome challenges, and ultimately achieve your weight loss goals.

Remember, weight loss isn't just about the number on the scale—it's about building a **healthier lifestyle** that allows you to live your life to the fullest. Celebrate your progress, lean on your support system, and stay true to your goals. You're not only changing your body—you're transforming your life, and that journey is always better when shared.

Chapter 8: The Science of Metabolism, Nutrition, and Behavior

8.1 Understanding Energy Balance and Metabolism

8.1.1 The Concept of Energy Balance

At the core of weight loss is the concept of **energy balance**, which refers to the relationship between **energy intake** (calories consumed through food and beverages) and **energy expenditure** (calories burned through physical activity, metabolic processes, and thermogenesis). Understanding how to manipulate energy balance is essential to achieving and maintaining weight loss.

- **Caloric Deficit**: To lose weight, a **caloric deficit** must be created—meaning that the number of calories you consume must be less than the number of calories you burn. This deficit forces the body to use stored fat as an energy source, leading to weight loss over time.

  - **Energy Intake and Quality**: While the quantity of calories is crucial, the **quality of calories** also plays an important role. **100 calories** from a sugary snack are not the same as **100 calories** from a nutrient-dense food like **vegetables or lean proteins.** The types of food you consume influence **satiety, metabolism**, and **nutritional health**, which ultimately impact your weight loss success.

- **Energy Expenditure Components**: Energy expenditure has three primary components:

  - **Basal Metabolic Rate (BMR)**: The number of calories your body needs to maintain basic physiological functions like breathing, circulation, and cell production. BMR accounts for **60-70%** of total daily energy expenditure.

  - **Physical Activity**: The calories burned through all forms of activity, including **exercise, work-related tasks**, and **daily movements** (such as walking or cleaning). This component is highly variable and can range from **20-30%** of energy expenditure.

  - **Thermic Effect of Food (TEF)**: The energy required to digest, absorb, and metabolize food. TEF makes up about **10%** of daily calorie expenditure, depending on the types of foods eaten (protein requires more energy to digest than fats or carbohydrates).

8.1.2 Basal Metabolic Rate and Factors That Affect It

Basal Metabolic Rate (BMR) is a key determinant of energy expenditure and varies significantly from person to person. Understanding what influences BMR can help you better understand why weight loss might be easier or more challenging for different individuals.

- **Genetics**: Genetics play a significant role in determining your BMR. Some individuals naturally have a higher BMR due to genetic factors, meaning they burn more calories at rest compared to others with a similar body size and composition.

- **Muscle Mass**: Muscle tissue is more metabolically active than fat tissue, meaning it burns more calories even at rest. Individuals with higher **muscle mass** tend to have a higher BMR. This is why **resistance training** is crucial for boosting BMR and promoting weight loss.

- **Age: BMR** generally decreases with age, which is partly due to a loss of muscle mass and changes in hormone levels. As people age, their caloric needs decrease, making it easier to gain weight if dietary habits are not adjusted.

- **Hormonal Influences**: Hormones such as **thyroid hormones (T3 and T4), cortisol,** and **sex hormones (estrogen and testosterone)** play important roles in regulating BMR. Thyroid dysfunction, for example, can lead to a decreased metabolic rate, making weight loss more challenging.

- **Gender: Men** typically have a higher BMR compared to **women** due to having a higher proportion of muscle mass and larger body size. However, muscle-building exercises can help women increase their BMR and improve weight loss outcomes.

8.1.3 Adaptive Thermogenesis and Metabolic Adaptation

Adaptive thermogenesis refers to the body's ability to adjust its metabolic rate in response to changes in energy intake or expenditure. This phenomenon is often observed during weight loss, where the body reduces its energy expenditure in response to a prolonged caloric deficit, making it harder to lose additional weight. This is an example of **metabolic adaptation**—the body's effort to maintain energy balance and prevent starvation.

- **Plateaus in Weight Loss: Metabolic adaptation** is one of the main reasons why individuals often experience **plateaus** during weight loss. When weight loss slows down despite maintaining a caloric deficit, it's often because the body has adjusted to the lower energy intake, and the BMR has decreased as a result.

- **How to Overcome Adaptive Thermogenesis**: To overcome metabolic adaptation, consider **cycling calories** through techniques such as **refeed days** (days with slightly higher calorie intake) or **reverse dieting** (gradually increasing calories after a period of restriction to boost metabolism). **Strength training** is also key to preserving or building muscle mass, which helps counteract the reduction in BMR that occurs with weight loss.

8.2 The Role of Macronutrients in Weight Loss

8.2.1 Understanding Macronutrients

Macronutrients are the nutrients required in large amounts and include **carbohydrates, proteins**, and **fats**. Each macronutrient plays a unique role in the body, and balancing these macronutrients is crucial for effective weight loss.

- **Carbohydrates**: Carbohydrates are the body's primary energy source. They are broken down into **glucose**, which fuels cells and supports physical activity. Carbs can be categorized into **simple** and **complex** carbohydrates. **Complex carbs** (such as whole grains, legumes, and vegetables) are rich in fiber and provide a slow, steady release of energy, which helps with satiety and blood sugar control.

- **Proteins: Protein** is essential for building and repairing tissues, including muscle. It also plays a significant role in satiety, as it takes longer to digest compared to carbohydrates and fats. A high-protein diet can help preserve **lean body mass** during weight loss, which is important for maintaining metabolic rate. Sources of protein include **lean meats, poultry, fish, eggs, dairy products, legumes**, and **plant-based protein sources** like tofu and tempeh.

- **Fats**: Dietary **fats** are essential for the absorption of fat-soluble vitamins (A, D, E, K), hormone production, and maintaining cell structure. Fats can be categorized into **saturated, monounsaturated,** and **polyunsaturated** fats. **Healthy fats** like **olive oil, avocados, nuts**, and **seeds** help provide satiety, making it easier to maintain a caloric deficit without feeling deprived.

8.2.2 Macronutrient Ratios for Weight Loss

The ratio of macronutrients can significantly impact weight loss, energy levels, and satiety. Different diets emphasize different macronutrient ratios, and finding the balance that works for you is essential.

- **High-Protein Diets: High-protein diets** are popular for weight loss due to their ability to increase satiety and preserve muscle mass during a caloric deficit. A diet that provides **25-30%** of total calories from protein can help reduce hunger, boost metabolism (due to the thermic effect of protein), and improve weight loss outcomes.

- **Low-Carbohydrate Diets: Low-carb diets** (such as the **keto diet** or **Atkins diet**) focus on reducing carbohydrate intake to promote fat metabolism. These diets encourage the body to enter a state of **ketosis**, where it uses **fat** as the primary fuel source. Low-carb diets can be effective for short-term weight loss, but sustainability is often a concern for many people. Additionally, it's important to ensure adequate nutrient intake when following a low-carb diet.

- **Balanced Diets:** A **balanced macronutrient approach** involves a moderate intake of carbohydrates, proteins, and fats, typically around **40-50% carbohydrates, 25-30% protein**, and **20-30% fat**. This type of diet is sustainable for most people and provides flexibility in food choices while ensuring nutrient needs are met.

8.2.3 The Role of Fiber in Weight Loss

Fiber is a type of carbohydrate that the body cannot fully digest, and it plays a significant role in weight management. Fiber-rich foods provide bulk, which helps with **satiety**, regulate **blood sugar levels**, and promote **digestive health**.

- **Soluble vs. Insoluble Fiber:** Fiber can be classified into **soluble** and **insoluble** types. **Soluble fiber** (found in foods like oats, beans, and fruits) dissolves in water to form a gel-like substance, which slows digestion and helps with fullness. **Insoluble fiber** (found in whole grains and vegetables) adds bulk to the stool and helps with regular bowel movements.

- **Increasing Fiber Intake:** Consuming more fiber can help control hunger and reduce overall calorie intake. Aim to include **fruits, vegetables, whole grains, legumes**, and **nuts** in your diet to meet the recommended daily fiber intake of **25-30 grams**. When increasing fiber, it's important to drink plenty of water to prevent digestive discomfort.

8.3 The Role of Micronutrients in Weight Loss

8.3.1 Importance of Micronutrients for Health and Weight Loss

Micronutrients—vitamins and minerals—are essential for maintaining **metabolic functions, immune health,** and **energy production**. While they don't directly contribute calories, they play vital roles in supporting weight loss.

- **Vitamins:** Certain vitamins, like the **B-complex vitamins (B6, B12, folate, niacin),** are crucial for **energy metabolism** and help the body convert food into energy. **Vitamin D** supports bone health, immune function, and may influence mood, which can affect eating behaviors.

- **Minerals: Minerals** like **iron, calcium, magnesium, and zinc** are essential for various physiological functions. **Iron** supports oxygen transport in the blood, which is vital for energy during physical activity. **Magnesium** plays a role in muscle function and stress management, while **zinc** helps with metabolism and immune function.

- **Electrolytes:** Electrolytes such as **sodium, potassium,** and **calcium** are important for maintaining fluid balance, nerve function, and muscle contractions. During exercise or when following certain diets (e.g., keto), electrolyte imbalances can occur, leading to symptoms like muscle cramps or fatigue. Maintaining a balance of electrolytes through diet or supplementation can enhance performance and support weight loss.

8.3.2 Common Micronutrient Deficiencies During Weight Loss

Weight loss diets can sometimes lead to **micronutrient deficiencies** if not well-balanced. Here are some common deficiencies and how to prevent them:

- **Calcium and Vitamin D**: Many individuals following a weight loss diet reduce their intake of dairy products, leading to lower calcium and vitamin D levels. To prevent deficiencies, include **leafy greens, fortified plant milks**, or consider taking a **vitamin D supplement** if needed.

- **Iron**: Reduced intake of **red meat** or inadequate consumption of iron-rich plant foods can lead to low iron levels, especially in women. Include iron-rich foods such as **lean meats, legumes, dark leafy greens**, and **fortified cereals** to maintain iron status. **Vitamin C** helps enhance iron absorption from plant sources, so pair iron-rich foods with vitamin C-rich foods (e.g., bell peppers, oranges).

- **Magnesium**: A deficiency in magnesium is common, especially for those on calorie-restricted diets. **Nuts, seeds, dark leafy greens, avocados**, and **whole grains** are excellent sources of magnesium. Including these foods helps support **muscle function, stress management**, and **sleep quality**.

8.4 The Gut Microbiome and Its Role in Weight Loss

8.4.1 Understanding the Gut Microbiome

The **gut microbiome** refers to the trillions of microorganisms, including bacteria, fungi, and viruses, that reside in the gastrointestinal tract. Recent research has shown that the gut microbiome plays a crucial role in **metabolism, immunity**, and even **weight regulation**.

- **Diversity of Gut Bacteria**: A diverse gut microbiome is linked to better health and more efficient metabolism. **Dysbiosis**, or an imbalance of gut bacteria, has been linked to obesity and metabolic disorders. Certain gut bacteria can extract more energy from food, potentially contributing to weight gain.

- **Influence on Appetite and Cravings**: The gut microbiome influences the production of hormones related to **appetite regulation**, such as **ghrelin** (the hunger hormone) and **leptin** (the satiety hormone). An imbalance in gut bacteria can lead to dysregulated hunger signals, increased cravings for sugar, and overeating.

8.4.2 Foods That Support a Healthy Gut Microbiome

- **Prebiotics: Prebiotics** are non-digestible fibers that promote the growth of beneficial gut bacteria. Foods rich in prebiotics include **bananas, onions, garlic, leeks, asparagus**, and **oats**. Including prebiotic foods in your diet helps feed the good bacteria in your gut, contributing to a more diverse and healthier microbiome.

- **Probiotics: Probiotics** are live bacteria that provide health benefits when consumed. Foods rich in probiotics include **yogurt, kefir, sauerkraut, kimchi**, and **miso**. Probiotics can help maintain a balance of gut bacteria and support digestion and immune function.

- **Diverse Diet for Diversity**: Eating a diverse diet rich in **fruits, vegetables, whole grains, legumes**, and **fermented foods** promotes gut microbial diversity. Each type of food provides different nutrients that support different strains of gut bacteria, making a varied diet key to a healthy microbiome.

8.4.3 The Gut-Brain Axis and Emotional Eating

The gut and brain communicate through the **gut-brain axis**, a bidirectional communication system involving the **nervous system, hormones**, and **immune system**. This connection plays a role in regulating mood, appetite, and behavior.

- **Gut Health and Mood**: The gut microbiome influences the production of **neurotransmitters** like **serotonin** (which regulates mood). An imbalance in the gut microbiome can impact mood and stress levels, which may lead to emotional eating.

Supporting gut health through diet can have a positive effect on mood and emotional regulation.

- **Mind-Gut Techniques**: Practicing **mindful eating, stress management techniques**, and consuming a diet that supports gut health can help reduce emotional eating. Techniques such as **meditation, deep breathing**, and **yoga** can help reduce stress and improve the gut-brain connection, supporting overall health and reducing overeating tendencies.

8.5 The Impact of Hormones on Weight Loss

8.5.1 Key Hormones Involved in Hunger and Satiety

Hormones play a significant role in regulating hunger, metabolism, and fat storage. Understanding the role of hormones can help you manage hunger and make more informed choices that support weight loss.

- **Leptin: Leptin** is known as the "satiety hormone." It is produced by fat cells and signals the brain to reduce appetite when energy stores are sufficient. Individuals with **obesity** often have higher leptin levels, but they may develop **leptin resistance,** where the brain does not receive the proper satiety signal, leading to overeating.

- **Ghrelin: Ghrelin** is known as the "hunger hormone." It is produced in the stomach and signals the brain to stimulate appetite. Ghrelin levels typically increase before meals and decrease afterward. High levels of ghrelin can make weight loss more challenging by increasing hunger.

- **Insulin: Insulin** is a hormone produced by the pancreas that helps regulate blood sugar levels. When carbohydrates are consumed, insulin is released to transport glucose into cells for energy or storage. **Insulin resistance** occurs when cells no longer respond effectively to insulin, leading to elevated blood sugar levels and increased fat storage.

8.5.2 Managing Hormones for Weight Loss

- **Balancing Meals:** Eating **balanced meals** that include **protein, healthy fats**, and **fiber** can help regulate insulin and blood sugar levels, keeping hunger hormones like ghrelin in check. Protein, in particular, has been shown to reduce ghrelin levels and promote satiety.

- **Prioritizing Sleep: Sleep** plays a significant role in regulating hormones related to hunger. **Poor sleep** has been linked to higher levels of ghrelin and lower levels of leptin, leading to increased hunger and cravings. Aim for **7-9 hours** of quality sleep per night to support hormone balance and weight management.

- **Managing Stress**: Chronic **stress** leads to elevated levels of **cortisol,** a hormone that can increase appetite and promote fat storage, particularly in the abdominal area. Incorporating **stress management practices** like **meditation, yoga,** or **deep breathing** can help reduce cortisol levels and improve weight loss outcomes.

8.6 Exploring Popular Diets: The Science Behind Them

8.6.1 Low-Carbohydrate Diets and the Ketogenic Diet

- **Low-Carb and Keto Diets: Low-carb diets** limit carbohydrate intake and emphasize proteins and fats, while **keto diets** are extremely low in carbohydrates, moderate in protein, and high in fat. The goal of the keto diet is to reach **ketosis,** where the body primarily uses **fat** as an energy source. These diets can be effective for weight loss in the short term and have shown benefits for **blood sugar regulation.**

- **Benefits and Challenges**: Low-carb diets can lead to rapid weight loss, particularly from reduced water retention. However, they can be challenging to sustain long-term, and some individuals may experience side effects like the "**keto flu**" (fatigue, headache, irritability). Long-term success depends on finding a balance and transitioning to a more sustainable way of eating.

8.6.2 Intermittent Fasting

- **How Intermittent Fasting Works: Intermittent fasting (IF)** involves alternating periods of eating and fasting. Popular approaches include the **16/8 method** (16 hours fasting, 8 hours eating) or **5:2 fasting** (eating normally for 5 days and restricting calories for 2 days). IF aims to create a caloric deficit, improve **insulin sensitivity**, and promote **autophagy** (cellular cleaning).

- **Benefits and Considerations**: IF can help some individuals reduce overall calorie intake and improve metabolic health. However, it is not suitable for everyone, especially those with a history of **eating disorders** or individuals who may have difficulty with extended fasting periods. Listening to your body and choosing an eating pattern that feels sustainable is crucial.

8.6.3 Plant-Based Diets

- **What is a Plant-Based Diet?**: A **plant-based diet** focuses on consuming mostly **fruits, vegetables, whole grains, legumes**, nuts, and seeds, with limited or no animal products. These diets are rich in **fiber, vitamins**, and **phytonutrients** that promote overall health.

- **Benefits for Weight Loss**: Plant-based diets are often lower in calorie density, which can make it easier to maintain a caloric deficit. The high fiber content also helps with satiety and digestive health. Studies have shown that individuals following plant-based diets tend to have lower body weight and reduced risk of chronic diseases.

- **Considerations for Nutrient Intake**: While plant-based diets offer many health benefits, it is important to ensure adequate intake of certain nutrients, such as **protein, vitamin B12, iron, omega-3 fatty acids**, and **calcium**. Including a variety of **plant proteins, fortified foods**, and **supplements** can help meet these needs.

8.6.4 The Mediterranean Diet

- **Overview**: The **Mediterranean diet** is based on the traditional eating patterns of countries bordering the Mediterranean Sea. It emphasizes **whole grains, vegetables, fruits, legumes, nuts, olive oil**, and **fish**, with moderate dairy and limited red meat.

- **Benefits for Weight Loss and Health**: The Mediterranean diet has been associated with numerous health benefits, including improved **cardiovascular health, weight loss**, and **reduced**

inflammation. It provides a balanced macronutrient ratio and promotes nutrient-dense foods, making it a sustainable and healthy option for long-term weight management.

- **Sustainable Lifestyle**: One of the main benefits of the Mediterranean diet is its emphasis on **enjoying food, social eating,** and **physical activity**. It is not a restrictive diet but a balanced approach that encourages variety and satisfaction.

8.6.5 Calorie Counting and Flexible Dieting

- **What is Flexible Dieting?: Flexible dieting**, also known as **"If It Fits Your Macros" (IIFYM)**, involves tracking **macronutrient intake** (protein, carbs, fat) and aiming to meet daily targets while allowing flexibility in food choices. It is a more individualized approach that emphasizes food freedom while staying within a caloric goal.

- **Benefits and Challenges**: Flexible dieting allows individuals to enjoy all foods in moderation, which can help with adherence and reduce feelings of deprivation. It requires a level of knowledge about food composition and portion sizes, which may be challenging for beginners. Tracking calories and macros can be effective, but it's also important to avoid becoming overly obsessed with numbers.

8.7 Behavioral Strategies for Long-Term Success

8.7.1 Understanding Behavior Change for Weight Loss

Behavior change is at the core of long-term weight management. To successfully lose weight and keep it off, it is important to understand the stages of behavior change and identify strategies that work for you.

- **Stages of Change Model**: The **Transtheoretical Model (TTM)**, or **Stages of Change Model**, outlines five stages of behavior change:

    1. **Precontemplation**: Not considering a change.

    2. **Contemplation**: Considering a change but not yet ready.

    3. **Preparation**: Getting ready to make a change.

    4. **Action**: Actively taking steps toward change.

    5. **Maintenance**: Sustaining the change over time.

Understanding where you are in this cycle can help you set appropriate goals and stay motivated.

- **Setting SMART Goals**: Effective goal setting involves creating **Specific, Measurable, Achievable, Relevant**, and **Time-bound (SMART)** goals. Instead of saying, "I want to lose weight," a SMART goal would be, "I will walk for 30 minutes every day after dinner for the next four weeks." This kind of goal is clear and provides a framework for success.

8.7.2 The Power of Habits and Daily Routines

Habits are automatic behaviors that are triggered by cues in our environment. Building positive habits and breaking negative ones is crucial for weight loss success.

- **The Habit Loop**: A habit loop consists of a **cue, routine**, and **reward**. For example, if stress (cue) leads to eating a snack (routine) for comfort (reward), it's important to replace the routine with a healthier one—such as **taking a walk or practicing deep breathing**—while still addressing the cue and getting a reward.

- **Building Healthy Habits**: Start small and build habits gradually. If your goal is to exercise regularly, start with **10-minute daily walks** and gradually increase the duration or intensity. Consistency is key—over time, these small changes will lead to lasting habits that support weight management.

8.7.3 Cognitive Behavioral Techniques for Weight Management

Cognitive Behavioral Therapy (CBT) is an effective approach to changing thought patterns and behaviors related to eating, exercise, and weight loss.

- **Identifying Cognitive Distortions: Cognitive distortions** are negative thought patterns that can hinder weight loss efforts. Examples include **all-or-nothing thinking** ("I ate one cookie, so I've ruined my diet") and **catastrophizing** ("I didn't work out today, so I'll never reach my goal"). Recognizing these patterns allows you to challenge and replace them with more realistic and positive thoughts.

- **Reframing Negative Thoughts**: Reframing negative thoughts involves turning a discouraging thought into a constructive one. For instance, if you think, "I'll never be able to lose weight," reframe it to, "I've faced challenges before, and I can learn to overcome this one too." Reframing helps build resilience and maintain motivation.

- **Mindful Eating Techniques: Mindful eating** involves paying full attention to the experience of eating—savoring flavors, noticing textures, and listening to hunger and fullness cues. Practicing mindful eating can help you develop a healthier relationship with food and reduce overeating.

8.7.4 Creating a Supportive Environment

A **supportive environment** is critical for long-term success in weight loss. This includes both the physical environment and the social support systems in your life.

- **Home Environment**: Create an environment that makes healthy choices easier. Keep **healthy foods** visible and accessible, while keeping treats out of sight or only bringing them into the house occasionally. Setting up a dedicated space for **physical activity** or exercise equipment can also encourage consistent activity.

- **Social Support**: Build a network of supportive friends, family, or online communities who understand and respect your goals. Having people who celebrate your successes and offer encouragement during setbacks helps keep you motivated.

- **Overcoming Triggers**: Identify triggers that lead to overeating or unhealthy behaviors and develop strategies to overcome them. For instance, if stress is a trigger, practice **stress-relief techniques** like **yoga, deep breathing**, or **journaling**. If boredom is a trigger, find alternative activities that keep you engaged, like **reading, walking**, or **crafting**.

8.8 The Science of Long-Term Weight Maintenance

8.8.1 Why Long-Term Maintenance is Challenging

While losing weight can be challenging, maintaining weight loss is often even more difficult due to the body's natural desire to return to its previous state, a phenomenon known as **"set point theory."** Understanding the science of weight maintenance can help overcome these challenges.

- **Set Point Theory**: The **set point theory** suggests that the body has a predetermined weight range that it "defends" through hormonal regulation. When weight is lost, the body may attempt to regain the weight through increased hunger and reduced energy expenditure. Consistently practicing healthy habits over time can help adjust the set point to a new, lower range.

- **Managing Adaptations**: After weight loss, adaptive mechanisms such as a slower metabolism and increased hunger can make maintenance challenging. Continuing **physical activity, resistance training,** and being mindful of portion sizes are critical strategies to counteract these changes and maintain weight loss.

8.8.2 Developing Resilience and Managing Relapse

Maintaining weight loss requires resilience and the ability to recover from setbacks. Understanding that lapses are a normal part of the process can help you stay on track without losing motivation.

- **Expecting and Planning for Lapses**: Lapses in diet or exercise habits are inevitable, especially during periods of high stress, holidays, or other life changes. Planning for these moments in advance and creating **"if-then"** strategies (e.g., "If I overeat at a party, then I'll focus on balanced meals the next day") can help you get back on track quickly.

- **Learning from Setbacks**: Setbacks can be valuable learning opportunities. Reflect on what led to a lapse and consider how to prevent similar situations in the future. Use these experiences as a way to improve your coping strategies and build resilience.

8.8.3 Sustainable Lifestyle Changes

Sustainable weight loss is about building a lifestyle that supports **health, balance**, and **enjoyment**. Drastic or restrictive approaches often lead to yo-yo dieting, which can be damaging both physically and emotionally.

- **Finding Enjoyable Activities**: Physical activity is essential for weight maintenance, but it doesn't have to mean spending hours in the gym. Find activities you enjoy—whether it's **dancing, hiking, biking**, or **yoga**. Enjoyment makes it easier to stick with regular physical activity long-term.

- **Balanced Eating**: Aim for **balance** in your diet, not perfection. Incorporate a variety of **nutrient-dense foods** while allowing for flexibility to enjoy treats in moderation. The 80/20 rule—where 80% of the time you focus on healthy choices and 20% of the time you allow for indulgences—can help maintain balance without feeling deprived.

- **Monitoring and Adapting**: Regularly **monitor your progress** to ensure you stay on track. Weighing yourself periodically, taking body measurements, or tracking habits in a journal can help you identify trends and make adjustments when needed. The goal isn't to be overly rigid but to be mindful and proactive about maintaining a healthy weight.

Chapter 9: The Psychology of Eating: Emotional and Behavioral Aspects of Weight Management

9.1 Understanding Emotional Eating

9.1.1 What is Emotional Eating?

Emotional eating is the tendency to eat in response to emotions rather than hunger. For many individuals, food becomes a coping mechanism to deal with emotions such as **stress, sadness, boredom, loneliness**, or even **happiness**. Emotional eating can lead to overeating and may hinder weight loss efforts by adding extra, unnecessary calories to one's daily intake.

- **Emotional vs. Physical Hunger**: One of the first steps in understanding emotional eating is learning to differentiate between **emotional hunger** and **physical hunger**. Emotional hunger comes on suddenly, is often tied to specific cravings (e.g., sweets, salty snacks), and is driven by feelings. Physical hunger, on the other hand, builds gradually, can be satisfied with a variety of foods, and is tied to the body's need for fuel.

- **Common Triggers for Emotional Eating**: Emotional eating is often triggered by specific emotions, situations, or stressors. Common triggers include **work stress, relationship problems, fatigue**, and even **social events**. Understanding what triggers emotional eating is the first step toward addressing it effectively.

- **Why Food Becomes a Coping Mechanism**: Food is easily accessible, comforting, and provides a quick mood boost, especially when high in **sugar** or **fat**, which release **dopamine** and create a sense of pleasure. Over time, these eating patterns become habitual, and individuals may begin to associate food with emotional relief, leading to the development of a conditioned response to emotional distress.

9.1.2 The Cycle of Emotional Eating

- **The Emotional Eating Cycle**: Emotional eating often leads to a cycle of **guilt, overeating, and restriction**. It begins with an emotional trigger, which leads to eating as a way to cope with the feeling. This eating is followed by guilt or shame, leading to more restrictive behaviors, which in turn can trigger further emotional eating.

- **Breaking the Cycle**: To break the cycle of emotional eating, it's important to replace food with healthier coping mechanisms. This involves identifying emotional triggers, practicing alternative behaviors, and learning to address the underlying emotions in a productive manner.

- **The Role of Guilt and Shame**: **Guilt** and **shame** are common feelings that follow emotional eating. Guilt comes from the behavior itself ("I shouldn't have eaten that"), while shame is related to identity ("I am weak for eating that"). These emotions can lead to further overeating as individuals attempt to soothe their negative feelings, perpetuating the cycle of emotional eating. Addressing guilt and practicing

self-compassion can help mitigate the negative emotional impact.

9.1.3 Types of Emotional Eating

Emotional eating can take on different forms, depending on the type of emotion involved and the individual's response to that emotion.

- **Stress Eating: Stress** is one of the most common triggers for emotional eating. During periods of stress, the body releases **cortisol**, a hormone that can increase appetite and cravings for high-calorie foods. The stress-eating response is often a way of self-soothing, as high-calorie foods can temporarily elevate mood by releasing endorphins.

- **Boredom Eating: Boredom** can also be a significant trigger for eating, as food provides a distraction and a temporary activity. People may find themselves reaching for snacks simply because there is nothing else to do or because eating provides a break from monotony.

- **Comfort Eating for Sadness or Loneliness**: For many, food becomes a source of comfort during times of **sadness or loneliness**. Foods that are associated with childhood, positive memories, or loved ones can bring about a temporary sense of connection or relief from negative feelings.

<h2 style="text-align:center">9.2 Exploring Food Addiction</h2>

<h3 style="text-align:center">9.2.1 Understanding Food Addiction</h3>

Food addiction is a concept used to describe an inability to resist certain foods, leading to compulsive eating behavior. Certain foods, especially those high in **sugar, fat**, and **salt,** can have similar effects on the brain as addictive substances like **drugs** or **alcohol**. These foods trigger the release of **dopamine**, which activates the brain's reward system and creates a desire for repeated consumption.

- **The Science Behind Food Addiction**: The concept of food addiction is supported by research into **neurotransmitters** and **brain chemistry**. When individuals consume highly palatable foods, the brain releases **dopamine** in the **nucleus accumbens**—an area associated with reward and pleasure. Over time, the brain may adapt to this overstimulation, requiring more of the food to achieve the same level of pleasure, similar to the way addiction to substances develops.

- **Signs and Symptoms of Food Addiction**: Symptoms of food addiction can include **cravings for certain foods, eating more than intended, eating despite negative consequences, loss of control** over eating, and **persistent desire** or **unsuccessful attempts** to cut down on eating certain foods. Emotional and physical symptoms of withdrawal, such as **irritability** or **anxiety,** may also occur when trying to abstain from trigger foods.

<h3 style="text-align:center">9.2.2 Identifying Trigger Foods and Behaviors</h3>

- **Highly Palatable Foods**: Foods that are highly processed, high in sugar, fat, and salt, are often referred to as **"hyper-palatable foods."** These foods are designed to be extremely rewarding and difficult to resist. Examples include **cookies, chips, ice cream**, and **fast food**. Identifying which foods trigger **compulsive eating** is a crucial first step in managing food addiction.

- **Situational Triggers**: In addition to certain foods, specific **situations** or **environments** can also trigger food cravings. For example, watching TV in the evening might be a trigger for snacking on chips, while visiting a particular friend could be associated with indulging in dessert. Identifying these situations helps in creating strategies to either avoid or manage them without overeating.

9.2.3 Overcoming Food Addiction

Overcoming food addiction requires a combination of **behavioral changes**, **emotional awareness**, and, in some cases, **professional help**. It involves developing new coping mechanisms and altering the relationship with food to reduce the addictive cycle.

- **Breaking the Reward Cycle**: The reward cycle of food addiction can be broken by reducing the frequency of consuming trigger foods. **Gradual reduction** is often more effective than complete elimination, as it helps reduce the intensity of cravings. By consistently choosing healthier alternatives, individuals can gradually shift the brain's reward system toward different, non-food-based rewards.

- **Behavioral Techniques**: Behavioral strategies such as **stimulus control** (removing trigger foods from the home) and **response substitution** (replacing the urge to eat with an alternative activity, such as going for a walk or drinking a glass of water) can help break the cycle of compulsive eating.

- **Seeking Professional Support**: In some cases, food addiction may require professional help from a **therapist, dietitian, or support group. Cognitive Behavioral Therapy (CBT), 12-step programs,** or **group counseling** can provide valuable support and tools for managing compulsive eating behaviors.

9.3 Developing Mindful Eating Practices

9.3.1 What is Mindful Eating?

Mindful eating is the practice of bringing full awareness to the act of eating—paying attention to the taste, texture, and experience of food while also being aware of hunger and satiety cues. It is about being present in the moment and eating without judgment.

- **The Core Principles of Mindful Eating**: The key principles of mindful eating include:

  - **Eating Slowly and Without Distraction**: Taking time to savor each bite and avoiding distractions like TV or smartphones while eating.

  - **Recognizing Hunger and Fullness Cues**: Eating when truly hungry and stopping when comfortably full, rather than eating out of habit or emotion.

  - **Engaging All Senses**: Paying attention to the colors, smells, tastes, and textures of food to enhance the eating experience.

  - **Non-Judgmental Awareness**: Avoiding judgment about what is being eaten, how much, or how quickly, and instead observing these behaviors with curiosity.

9.3.2 Benefits of Mindful Eating for Weight Loss

- **Improved Satiety**: One of the most significant benefits of mindful eating is improved **satiety**. By eating slowly and paying attention to hunger and fullness cues, individuals are better able to recognize when they are full, reducing the likelihood of overeating.

- **Reduced Emotional Eating**: Mindful eating can also help reduce emotional eating by increasing awareness of the underlying emotions driving food choices. Instead of automatically reaching for food when feeling stressed or sad, individuals learn to pause, assess their feelings, and choose whether food is the best way to address them.

- **Enhanced Enjoyment of Food**: By savoring each bite, mindful eating can lead to greater enjoyment of food. This enhanced satisfaction can help reduce cravings for highly processed foods, as the focus shifts to appreciating the quality and taste of what is being eaten.

9.3.3 Strategies for Practicing Mindful Eating

- **Mindful Eating Exercises**: Practicing mindful eating exercises can help develop the skill of eating with awareness. One exercise is the **raisin exercise**, in which individuals spend several minutes observing a single raisin—looking at its texture, feeling its weight, smelling it, and then slowly eating it while paying attention to the entire experience.

- **Eating Without Distractions**: Set aside dedicated time for meals, free from distractions like phones, computers, or TV. Eating without distractions allows for greater awareness of the food and more conscious decision-making.

- **Check-In Before and During Eating**: Before eating, pause and ask yourself, **"Am I physically hungry?"** During the meal, pause halfway through and check in with your fullness level. This helps determine whether to continue eating or stop. Practicing these check-ins helps develop a deeper awareness of the body's signals.

9.4 Cognitive Behavioral Strategies for Behavior Change

9.4.1 Introduction to Cognitive Behavioral Therapy (CBT)

Cognitive Behavioral Therapy (CBT) is a type of therapy that focuses on identifying and changing **negative thought patterns** and **behaviors.** In the context of weight management, CBT can help individuals develop healthier eating behaviors, challenge self-defeating thoughts, and set realistic goals.

- **The CBT Model:** The **CBT model** is based on the idea that **thoughts, feelings,** and **behaviors** are interconnected. By changing negative or distorted thoughts, individuals can positively impact their emotions and behaviors, leading to healthier outcomes.

- **Application to Weight Management:** In weight management, CBT is used to address **emotional eating, negative body image, unhelpful eating habits,** and **self-sabotaging thoughts.** It provides practical tools to identify and challenge these issues, promoting lasting behavior change.

9.4.2 Identifying Cognitive Distortions Related to Eating

Cognitive distortions are irrational thought patterns that can lead to unhealthy behaviors and emotions. Identifying and challenging these distortions is a key component of CBT.

- **All-or-Nothing Thinking: All-or-nothing thinking** occurs when individuals view situations in black-and-white terms. For example, eating one "off-plan" food may lead to the thought, "I've ruined my diet; I may as well keep eating poorly." This type of thinking often leads to cycles of **binge eating** and **restriction**.

- **Catastrophizing: Catastrophizing** involves imagining the worst possible outcome, such as believing that one mistake will lead to complete failure. For example, "I skipped my workout today, which means I'll never be able to lose weight."

- **Labeling: Labeling** involves assigning negative labels to oneself, such as "I'm weak" or "I'm a failure." This type of thinking can undermine motivation and lead to feelings of **shame** and **hopelessness**, making it harder to stay on track.

9.4.3 Challenging Negative Thoughts

- **Thought Records:** A useful tool in CBT is the **thought record**. In a thought record, individuals write down the situation, the thoughts they had, how they felt, and the behaviors that followed. This process helps identify patterns of negative thinking and understand how thoughts affect feelings and actions.

- **Cognitive Restructuring: Cognitive restructuring** involves identifying negative thoughts and replacing them with more balanced, realistic thoughts. For example, instead of thinking, "I ate dessert, so I've ruined my diet," a more balanced thought might be, "One dessert doesn't ruin my progress. I can make a healthier choice at my next meal."

- **Behavioral Experiments: Behavioral experiments** are designed to test the validity of negative thoughts. For example, if an individual has the thought, "I can't control myself around sweets," a behavioral experiment might involve putting themselves in a situation where sweets are present while practicing mindful eating to test whether they can, in fact, control their intake.

9.5 Coping with Stress, Anxiety, and Depression

9.5.1 The Impact of Stress, Anxiety, and Depression on Eating Behavior

Stress, anxiety, and **depression** are common mental health conditions that significantly impact eating behavior. Understanding how these emotions influence eating can help individuals develop healthier coping strategies.

- **Stress and Cortisol: Chronic stress** leads to elevated levels of **cortisol**, which increases appetite, particularly for high-calorie, sugary foods. This is a survival mechanism, as the body interprets stress as a need for additional energy to handle a perceived threat. The result is often **stress eating**, which can hinder weight loss efforts.

- **Anxiety and Eating Patterns**: Anxiety can lead to changes in eating patterns, with some individuals eating more as a form of self-soothing and others eating less due to **loss of appetite**. Both extremes can affect weight management efforts.

- **Depression and Emotional Eating: Depression** can lead to increased **emotional eating,** particularly for comfort foods that are high in fat and sugar. For some, depression may also result in **loss of interest** in food and decreased appetite. Both overconsumption and underconsumption can be problematic for maintaining a healthy relationship with food.

9.5.2 Healthy Coping Mechanisms for Emotional Regulation

Developing **healthy coping mechanisms** for managing stress, anxiety, and depression is essential for weight management. When emotions are regulated in a healthier way, the need to turn to food as a coping mechanism is reduced.

- **Relaxation Techniques**: Techniques such as **deep breathing, progressive muscle relaxation**, and **guided imagery** can help reduce the body's stress response. Practicing these techniques regularly can reduce cortisol levels and alleviate stress-related eating.

- **Physical Activity: Exercise** is one of the most effective ways to manage stress, anxiety, and depression. It releases **endorphins**, which improve mood, reduce anxiety, and boost energy. Whether it's a **walk in nature, yoga session,** or **dance class,** physical activity can serve as a positive coping mechanism.

- **Mindfulness and Meditation: Mindfulness meditation** helps individuals become more aware of their thoughts and emotions without judgment. By practicing mindfulness regularly, individuals can develop a greater ability to tolerate uncomfortable emotions without reacting impulsively (e.g., overeating).

- **Creative Outlets**: Engaging in **creative activities,** such as **painting, writing, playing an instrument,** or **crafting,** can help process emotions and reduce stress. Creativity provides an outlet for emotions and is an effective way to cope with anxiety or low mood without turning to food.

9.5.3 Seeking Professional Help

When emotional challenges like **stress, anxiety,** or **depression** are overwhelming or persistent, seeking professional help is important. **Therapists, counselors,** and **mental health professionals** can provide tools and support for managing emotions in a healthy way.

- **Counseling and Therapy: Individual therapy**, such as **CBT**, can help address the underlying causes of emotional eating and provide tools for coping. **Group therapy** or **support groups** also offer a sense of community and support from others who are experiencing similar challenges.

- **Medication**: In some cases, medication may be necessary to manage conditions like **anxiety** or **depression**. A healthcare professional can evaluate whether medication is appropriate and provide guidance on its use. It's important to recognize that medication can be a valuable part of treatment, and there should be no stigma attached to seeking the help needed to feel well.

9.6 Building Resilience and Emotional Strength

9.6.1 What is Resilience?

Resilience is the ability to **bounce back** from setbacks, challenges, or difficult experiences. In the context of weight management, resilience is crucial because the journey often involves obstacles, such as **plateaus, emotional eating episodes**, or **social pressure.**

- **Characteristics of Resilient Individuals**: Resilient individuals tend to be **adaptable**, have a **positive** outlook, are **solution-focused**, and view challenges as opportunities for growth. Resilience is not an innate quality but a skill that can be cultivated through practice.

9.6.2 Developing a Growth Mindset

- **Growth vs. Fixed Mindset**: A **growth mindset** involves believing that abilities and qualities can be developed through effort and learning, whereas a **fixed mindset** involves seeing abilities as unchangeable. In weight management, a growth mindset means viewing setbacks as opportunities to learn and improve, rather than as failures.

- **Challenging Limiting Beliefs: Limiting beliefs** are negative thoughts that prevent progress, such as "I can't lose weight" or "I'll always be overweight." Challenging these beliefs by asking, "Is this thought true?" or "What evidence do I have to support this?" can help reframe them in a more positive light. Replacing limiting beliefs with **affirmations** like "I am capable of change" or "Every effort I make is a step forward" fosters a growth mindset.

9.6.3 Learning from Setbacks

Setbacks are an inevitable part of any journey, including weight loss. How you respond to setbacks determines whether you can overcome them and continue moving forward.

- **Analyzing Setbacks Without Judgment**: When experiencing a setback, take time to **analyze** it without self-judgment. Ask yourself, "What led to this situation?" "What can I learn from it?" and "What can I do differently next time?" This reflection helps identify areas for improvement without being overly critical.

- **Using Setbacks as Opportunities for Growth**: Reframing setbacks as opportunities for growth allows you to take a proactive approach to challenges. For example, if emotional eating occurs after a stressful day, consider how to better manage stress in the future—such as through **deep breathing, journaling**, or **reaching out to a friend**.

9.6.4 Practicing Self-Compassion

Self-compassion involves treating yourself with **kindness** and **understanding**, especially during times of struggle or failure. Many individuals who struggle with weight have a tendency to be harshly critical of themselves, but this often leads to feelings of guilt and shame, which can perpetuate unhealthy behaviors.

- **Three Components of Self-Compassion**: According to psychologist **Kristin Neff**, self-compassion has three components:

  - **Self-Kindness**: Being gentle and understanding with yourself, rather than harsh or self-critical.

- o **Common Humanity**: Recognizing that everyone makes mistakes and experiences difficulties; you are not alone.

- o **Mindfulness**: Being present with your feelings without over-identifying with them. Acknowledge negative emotions, but don't let them define you.

- **Self-Compassion Practices**: Practice **self-compassion** by speaking to yourself the way you would speak to a friend. When you experience a setback, ask yourself, "What would I say to a friend in this situation?" Write yourself a **compassionate letter** when you're struggling or repeat affirmations like, "I am doing my best, and that's enough."

9.7 Nurturing a Positive Body Image

9.7.1 Understanding Body Image

Body image is the perception of one's own body and how one feels about their physical appearance. It is influenced by a variety of factors, including **societal ideals, media, family**, and **peers**. Developing a positive body image is crucial for emotional well-being and sustainable weight management.

- **Negative Body Image: Negative body image** involves dissatisfaction with one's appearance, preoccupation with perceived flaws, and comparison to unrealistic standards. Negative body image is associated with **low self-esteem, depression**, and **disordered eating behaviors.**

- **Positive Body Image: Positive body image** means accepting, appreciating, and respecting your body as it is, regardless of its shape or size. It involves focusing on what your body can do and recognizing your worth beyond physical appearance.

9.7.2 Factors That Influence Body Image

- **Media and Societal Ideals**: Media often portrays a narrow and unrealistic standard of beauty that can impact body image. **Social media**, in particular, contributes to negative body image through **filtered** and **edited** images. Understanding that these images are not realistic representations helps reduce the pressure to conform to these ideals.

- **Family and Peer Influences**: Comments from **family** and **peers** about weight, appearance, or eating habits can also shape body image. **Positive role models** and **supportive family environments** can foster body appreciation, while negative comments can contribute to body dissatisfaction.

- **Comparison: Social comparison** is another significant factor in shaping body image. Constantly comparing oneself to others, especially in terms of weight or appearance, can lead to body dissatisfaction. Recognizing that every individual has a unique body and journey can help reduce the urge to compare.

9.7.3 Strategies for Building a Positive Body Image

- **Practice Body Neutrality: Body neutrality** involves focusing on what the body can do rather than how it looks. It is about appreciating your body for its strength, health, and capabilities, rather than its physical appearance. For example, instead of focusing on whether your legs look a certain way, focus on their ability to carry you through a **run, dance**, or **hike**.

- **Limit Exposure to Negative Influences**: Curate your **social media feed** to include accounts that promote **body positivity, diverse body types**, and **self-acceptance**. Unfollow accounts that make you feel bad about your body or promote unrealistic ideals.

- **Affirmations and Positive Self-Talk**: Use positive affirmations to counter negative thoughts about your body. Affirmations like "My body is strong," "I am grateful for my body," or "I deserve to take up space" can help shift focus from criticism to appreciation.

- **Dress for Comfort and Confidence**: Wearing clothes that make you feel comfortable and confident can have a significant impact on body image. Avoid clothing that feels restrictive or makes you self-conscious. Instead, choose outfits that fit well, are comfortable, and reflect your personal style.

9.8 Changing Your Relationship with Food

9.8.1 Moving Away from Diet Culture

Diet culture is the belief system that equates thinness with health and worthiness. It promotes **restriction, weight loss**, and **body control** as a way to achieve happiness and success. Moving away from diet culture involves challenging these beliefs and embracing a more balanced, sustainable approach to health and weight management.

- **Rejecting the "Good vs. Bad" Food Mentality**: One of the hallmarks of diet culture is labeling foods as **"good"** or **"bad."** This can lead to feelings of guilt when eating certain foods, which may lead to restriction or bingeing. Instead, aim to view food as **neutral**—recognize that all foods can fit into a healthy diet and that balance is key.

- **Focusing on Health, Not Weight**: Health is not solely determined by body weight. It is influenced by a variety of factors, including **mental well-being, physical activity, stress management**, and **balanced nutrition**. Shifting the focus away from weight and toward overall health helps develop a more positive relationship with both food and body.

- **Ditching the Scale**: Constantly weighing oneself can lead to fixation on a number rather than focusing on overall well-being. Consider **ditching the scale** or reducing the frequency of weigh-ins. Instead, monitor progress through **non-scale victories** such as increased energy, improved mood, better sleep, or clothing fitting differently.

9.8.2 Developing Food Freedom

Food freedom is the concept of being able to make food choices without feelings of guilt or fear. It involves allowing yourself to enjoy all foods in moderation and trusting your body to guide you.

- **Allowing All Foods**: Restrictive diets often lead to intense cravings and bingeing once the restriction ends. Instead, allow yourself to enjoy **all types of food**. When no food is off-limits, the urgency to overeat it is reduced. Learning to eat in moderation rather than complete avoidance helps build a balanced relationship with food.

- **Listening to Hunger and Fullness Cues**: Trusting and listening to your body's **hunger** and **fullness** cues is central to food freedom. Avoid eating based on arbitrary rules or schedules; instead, pay attention to your body's natural signals and eat when you're hungry and stop when you're full.

- **Satisfying Cravings Without Guilt**: Cravings are normal, and satisfying them in moderation is part of developing a healthy relationship with food. For example, if you're craving chocolate, have a piece of chocolate and savor it mindfully. When cravings are satisfied without guilt, the cycle of deprivation and bingeing is reduced.

9.8.3 Intuitive Eating as an Approach

Intuitive eating is an approach to eating that encourages individuals to trust their body's signals for hunger, fullness, and satisfaction. It was developed by **Evelyn Tribole** and **Elyse Resch** as an antidote to diet culture and emphasizes a positive relationship with food.

- **The Ten Principles of Intuitive Eating**: The ten principles of intuitive eating include:

  - **Rejecting Diet Mentality**: Letting go of the belief that there is a perfect diet that will lead to happiness and success.

  - **Honoring Your Hunger**: Eating when you are hungry to avoid extreme hunger, which can lead to overeating.

  - **Making Peace with Food**: Giving yourself unconditional permission to eat all foods without guilt.

  - **Challenging the Food Police**: Rejecting thoughts that label foods as "good" or "bad" or criticize your eating choices.

  - **Feeling Your Fullness**: Learning to recognize when you are comfortably full and satisfied.

- o **Discovering Satisfaction**: Eating what you truly want and savoring the experience can lead to greater satisfaction with less food.

  - o **Coping with Emotions Without Using Food**: Finding ways to cope with emotions that do not involve eating.

  - o **Respecting Your Body**: Accepting your body for what it is, rather than trying to change it to fit societal ideals.

  - o **Movement—Feel the Difference**: Focusing on the way movement makes you feel rather than just as a means to burn calories.

  - o **Honoring Your Health**: Choosing foods that honor your health and taste good, without rigid rules.

- **The Benefits of Intuitive Eating**: Research shows that intuitive eating is associated with **lower BMI**, **better psychological health**, and **reduced disordered eating behaviors**. It allows individuals to enjoy food without restriction, promoting long-term health and well-being.

9.9 Conclusion: The Emotional and Behavioral Keys to Weight Management Success

The psychology of eating is a complex, multifaceted aspect of weight management. Understanding the emotional and behavioral components of eating is crucial for developing a healthy, sustainable approach to weight loss. Emotional eating, food addiction, negative body image, and the pressures of diet culture are all challenges that can stand in the way of successful weight management.

By addressing the **emotional triggers** of eating, challenging **negative thoughts**, practicing **mindful eating**, building **resilience**, and nurturing a **positive body image**, individuals can transform their relationship with food and body. The goal is to move away from restriction, guilt, and self-criticism and toward **balance, compassion**, and **self-acceptance**.

Weight management is not just about what you eat; it's about why and how you eat. By focusing on the emotional and behavioral aspects of eating, you can develop the tools necessary to maintain weight loss, enjoy food without guilt, and live a healthier, more fulfilling life.

Chapter 9: The Psychology of Eating: Emotional and Behavioral Aspects of Weight Management

9.1 Understanding Emotional Eating

9.1.1 What is Emotional Eating?

Emotional eating is the tendency to eat in response to emotions rather than hunger. For many individuals, food becomes a coping mechanism to deal with emotions such as **stress, sadness, boredom, loneliness**, or even **happiness**. Emotional eating can lead to overeating and may hinder weight loss efforts by adding extra, unnecessary calories to one's daily intake.

- **Emotional vs. Physical Hunger**: One of the first steps in understanding emotional eating is learning to differentiate between **emotional hunger** and **physical hunger**. Emotional hunger comes on suddenly, is often tied to specific cravings (e.g., sweets, salty snacks), and is driven by feelings. Physical hunger, on the other hand, builds gradually, can be satisfied with a variety of foods, and is tied to the body's need for fuel.

- **Common Triggers for Emotional Eating**: Emotional eating is often triggered by specific emotions, situations, or stressors. Common triggers include **work stress, relationship problems, fatigue**, and even **social events**. Understanding what triggers emotional eating is the first step toward addressing it effectively.

- **Why Food Becomes a Coping Mechanism**: Food is easily accessible, comforting, and provides a quick mood boost, especially when high in **sugar** or **fat**, which release **dopamine** and create a sense of pleasure. Over time, these eating patterns become habitual, and individuals may begin to associate food with emotional relief, leading to the development of a conditioned response to emotional distress.

9.1.2 The Cycle of Emotional Eating

- **The Emotional Eating Cycle**: Emotional eating often leads to a cycle of **guilt, overeating, and restriction**. It begins with an emotional trigger, which leads to eating as a way to cope with the feeling. This eating is followed by guilt or shame, leading to more restrictive behaviors, which in turn can trigger further emotional eating.

- **Breaking the Cycle**: To break the cycle of emotional eating, it's important to replace food with healthier coping mechanisms. This involves identifying emotional triggers, practicing alternative behaviors, and learning to address the underlying emotions in a productive manner.

- **The Role of Guilt and Shame**: **Guilt** and **shame** are common feelings that follow emotional eating. Guilt comes from the behavior itself ("I shouldn't have eaten that"), while shame is related to identity ("I am weak for eating that"). These emotions can lead to further overeating as individuals attempt to soothe their negative feelings, perpetuating the cycle of emotional eating. Addressing guilt and practicing **self-compassion** can help mitigate the negative emotional impact.

9.1.3 Types of Emotional Eating

Emotional eating can take on different forms, depending on the type of emotion involved and the individual's response to that emotion.

- **Stress Eating: Stress** is one of the most common triggers for emotional eating. During periods of stress, the body releases **cortisol**, a hormone that can increase appetite and cravings for high-calorie foods. The stress-eating response is often a way of self-soothing, as high-calorie foods can temporarily elevate mood by releasing endorphins.

- **Boredom Eating: Boredom** can also be a significant trigger for eating, as food provides a distraction and a temporary activity. People may find themselves reaching for snacks simply because there is nothing else to do or because eating provides a break from monotony.

- **Comfort Eating for Sadness or Loneliness**: For many, food becomes a source of comfort during times of **sadness or loneliness**. Foods that are associated with childhood, positive memories, or loved ones can bring about a temporary sense of connection or relief from negative feelings.

9.2 Exploring Food Addiction

9.2.1 Understanding Food Addiction

Food addiction is a concept used to describe an inability to resist certain foods, leading to compulsive eating behavior. Certain foods, especially those high in **sugar, fat**, and **salt**, can have similar effects on the brain as addictive substances like **drugs** or **alcohol**. These foods trigger the release of **dopamine**, which activates the brain's reward system and creates a desire for repeated consumption.

- **The Science Behind Food Addiction**: The concept of food addiction is supported by research into **neurotransmitters** and **brain chemistry**. When individuals consume highly palatable foods, the brain releases **dopamine** in the **nucleus accumbens**—an area associated with reward and pleasure. Over time, the brain may adapt to this overstimulation, requiring more of the food to achieve the same level of pleasure, similar to the way addiction to substances develops.

- **Signs and Symptoms of Food Addiction**: Symptoms of food addiction can include **cravings for certain foods, eating more than intended, eating despite negative consequences, loss of control** over eating, and **persistent desire** or **unsuccessful attempts** to cut down on eating certain foods. Emotional and physical symptoms of withdrawal, such as **irritability** or **anxiety**, may also occur when trying to abstain from trigger foods.

9.2.2 Identifying Trigger Foods and Behaviors

- **Highly Palatable Foods**: Foods that are highly processed, high in sugar, fat, and salt, are often referred to as **"hyper-palatable foods."** These foods are designed to be extremely rewarding and difficult to resist. Examples include **cookies, chips, ice cream**, and **fast food**. Identifying which foods trigger **compulsive eating** is a crucial first step in managing food addiction.

- **Situational Triggers**: In addition to certain foods, specific **situations** or **environments** can also trigger food cravings. For example, watching TV in the evening might be a trigger for snacking on chips, while visiting a particular friend could be associated with indulging in dessert. Identifying these situations helps in creating strategies to either avoid or manage them without overeating.

9.2.3 Overcoming Food Addiction

Overcoming food addiction requires a combination of **behavioral changes, emotional awareness**, and, in some cases, **professional help**. It involves developing new coping mechanisms and altering the relationship with food to reduce the addictive cycle.

- **Breaking the Reward Cycle**: The reward cycle of food addiction can be broken by reducing the frequency of consuming trigger foods. **Gradual reduction** is often more effective than complete elimination, as it helps reduce the intensity of cravings. By consistently choosing healthier alternatives, individuals can gradually shift the brain's reward system toward different, non-food-based rewards.

- **Behavioral Techniques**: Behavioral strategies such as **stimulus control** (removing trigger foods from the home) and **response substitution** (replacing the urge to eat with an alternative activity, such as going for a walk or drinking a glass of water) can help break the cycle of compulsive eating.

- **Seeking Professional Support**: In some cases, food addiction may require professional help from a **therapist, dietitian, or support group. Cognitive Behavioral Therapy (CBT), 12-step programs**, or **group counseling** can provide valuable support and tools for managing compulsive eating behaviors.

9.3 Developing Mindful Eating Practices

9.3.1 What is Mindful Eating?

Mindful eating is the practice of bringing full awareness to the act of eating—paying attention to the taste, texture, and experience of food while also being aware of hunger and satiety cues. It is about being present in the moment and eating without judgment.

- **The Core Principles of Mindful Eating**: The key principles of mindful eating include:

  - **Eating Slowly and Without Distraction**: Taking time to savor each bite and avoiding distractions like TV or smartphones while eating.

  - **Recognizing Hunger and Fullness Cues**: Eating when truly hungry and stopping when comfortably full, rather than eating out of habit or emotion.

o   **Engaging All Senses**: Paying attention to the colors, smells, tastes, and textures of food to enhance the eating experience.

o   **Non-Judgmental Awareness**: Avoiding judgment about what is being eaten, how much, or how quickly, and instead observing these behaviors with curiosity.

9.3.2 Benefits of Mindful Eating for Weight Loss

- **Improved Satiety**: One of the most significant benefits of mindful eating is improved **satiety**. By eating slowly and paying attention to hunger and fullness cues, individuals are better able to recognize when they are full, reducing the likelihood of overeating.

- **Reduced Emotional Eating**: Mindful eating can also help reduce emotional eating by increasing awareness of the underlying emotions driving food choices. Instead of automatically reaching for food when feeling stressed or sad, individuals learn to pause, assess their feelings, and choose whether food is the best way to address them.

- **Enhanced Enjoyment of Food**: By savoring each bite, mindful eating can lead to greater enjoyment of food. This enhanced satisfaction can help reduce cravings for highly processed foods, as the focus shifts to appreciating the quality and taste of what is being eaten.

9.3.3 Strategies for Practicing Mindful Eating

- **Mindful Eating Exercises**: Practicing mindful eating exercises can help develop the skill of eating with awareness. One exercise is the **raisin exercise**, in which individuals spend several minutes observing a single raisin—looking at its texture, feeling its weight, smelling it, and then slowly eating it while paying attention to the entire experience.

- **Eating Without Distractions**: Set aside dedicated time for meals, free from distractions like phones, computers, or TV. Eating without distractions allows for greater awareness of the food and more conscious decision-making.

- **Check-In Before and During Eating**: Before eating, pause and ask yourself, **"Am I physically hungry?"** During the meal, pause halfway through and check in with your fullness level. This helps determine whether to continue eating or stop. Practicing these check-ins helps develop a deeper awareness of the body's signals.

9.4 Cognitive Behavioral Strategies for Behavior Change

9.4.1 Introduction to Cognitive Behavioral Therapy (CBT)

Cognitive Behavioral Therapy (CBT) is a type of therapy that focuses on identifying and changing **negative thought patterns** and **behaviors**. In the context of weight management, CBT can help individuals develop healthier eating behaviors, challenge self-defeating thoughts, and set realistic goals.

- **The CBT Model:** The **CBT model** is based on the idea that **thoughts, feelings,** and **behaviors** are interconnected. By changing negative or distorted thoughts, individuals can positively impact their emotions and behaviors, leading to healthier outcomes.

- **Application to Weight Management:** In weight management, CBT is used to address **emotional eating, negative body image, unhelpful eating habits,** and **self-sabotaging thoughts**. It provides practical tools to identify and challenge these issues, promoting lasting behavior change.

9.4.2 Identifying Cognitive Distortions Related to Eating

Cognitive distortions are irrational thought patterns that can lead to unhealthy behaviors and emotions. Identifying and challenging these distortions is a key component of CBT.

- **All-or-Nothing Thinking: All-or-nothing thinking** occurs when individuals view situations in black-and-white terms. For example, eating one "off-plan" food may lead to the thought, "I've ruined my diet; I may as well keep eating poorly." This type of thinking often leads to cycles of **binge eating** and **restriction**.

- **Catastrophizing: Catastrophizing** involves imagining the worst possible outcome, such as believing that one mistake will lead to complete failure. For example, "I skipped my workout today, which means I'll never be able to lose weight."

- **Labeling: Labeling** involves assigning negative labels to oneself, such as "I'm weak" or "I'm a failure." This type of thinking can undermine motivation and lead to feelings of **shame** and **hopelessness**, making it harder to stay on track.

9.4.3 Challenging Negative Thoughts

- **Thought Records**: A useful tool in CBT is the **thought record**. In a thought record, individuals write down the situation, the thoughts they had, how they felt, and the behaviors that followed. This process helps identify patterns of negative thinking and understand how thoughts affect feelings and actions.

- **Cognitive Restructuring: Cognitive restructuring** involves identifying negative thoughts and replacing them with more balanced, realistic thoughts. For example, instead of thinking, "I ate dessert, so I've ruined my diet," a more balanced thought might be, "One dessert doesn't ruin my progress. I can make a healthier choice at my next meal."

- **Behavioral Experiments: Behavioral experiments** are designed to test the validity of negative thoughts. For example, if an individual has the thought, "I can't control myself around sweets," a behavioral experiment might involve putting themselves in a situation where sweets are present while practicing mindful eating to test whether they can, in fact, control their intake.

9.5 Coping with Stress, Anxiety, and Depression

9.5.1 The Impact of Stress, Anxiety, and Depression on Eating Behavior

Stress, anxiety, and **depression** are common mental health conditions that significantly impact eating behavior. Understanding how these emotions influence eating can help individuals develop healthier coping strategies.

- **Stress and Cortisol: Chronic stress** leads to elevated levels of **cortisol**, which increases appetite, particularly for high-calorie, sugary foods. This is a survival mechanism, as the body interprets stress as a need for additional energy to handle a perceived threat. The result is often **stress eating**, which can hinder weight loss efforts.

- **Anxiety and Eating Patterns**: Anxiety can lead to changes in eating patterns, with some individuals eating more as a form of self-soothing and others eating less due to **loss of appetite**. Both extremes can affect weight management efforts.

- **Depression and Emotional Eating: Depression** can lead to increased **emotional eating**, particularly for comfort foods that are high in fat and sugar. For some, depression may also result in **loss of interest** in food and decreased appetite. Both overconsumption and underconsumption can be problematic for maintaining a healthy relationship with food.

9.5.2 Healthy Coping Mechanisms for Emotional Regulation

Developing **healthy coping mechanisms** for managing stress, anxiety, and depression is essential for weight management. When emotions are regulated in a healthier way, the need to turn to food as a coping mechanism is reduced.

- **Relaxation Techniques**: Techniques such as **deep breathing, progressive muscle relaxation**, and **guided imagery** can help reduce the body's stress response. Practicing these techniques regularly can reduce cortisol levels and alleviate stress-related eating.

- **Physical Activity: Exercise** is one of the most effective ways to manage stress, anxiety, and depression. It releases **endorphins**, which improve mood, reduce anxiety, and boost energy. Whether it's a **walk in nature, yoga session**, or **dance class**, physical activity can serve as a positive coping mechanism.

- **Mindfulness and Meditation: Mindfulness meditation** helps individuals become more aware of their thoughts and emotions without judgment. By practicing mindfulness regularly, individuals can develop a greater ability to tolerate uncomfortable emotions without reacting impulsively (e.g., overeating).

- **Creative Outlets**: Engaging in **creative activities**, such as **painting, writing, playing an instrument**, or **crafting**, can help process emotions and reduce stress. Creativity provides an outlet for emotions and is an effective way to cope with anxiety or low mood without turning to food.

9.5.3 Seeking Professional Help

When emotional challenges like **stress, anxiety**, or **depression** are overwhelming or persistent, seeking professional help is important. **Therapists, counselors**, and **mental health professionals** can provide tools and support for managing emotions in a healthy way.

- **Counseling and Therapy: Individual therapy**, such as **CBT**, can help address the underlying causes of emotional eating and provide tools for coping. **Group therapy** or **support groups** also offer a sense of community and support from others who are experiencing similar challenges.

- **Medication**: In some cases, medication may be necessary to manage conditions like **anxiety** or **depression**. A healthcare professional can evaluate whether medication is appropriate and provide guidance on its use. It's important to recognize that medication can be a valuable part of treatment, and there should be no stigma attached to seeking the help needed to feel well.

9.6 Building Resilience and Emotional Strength

9.6.1 What is Resilience?

Resilience is the ability to **bounce back** from setbacks, challenges, or difficult experiences. In the context of weight management, resilience is crucial because the journey often involves obstacles, such as **plateaus, emotional eating episodes,** or **social pressure**.

- **Characteristics of Resilient Individuals**: Resilient individuals tend to be **adaptable**, have a **positive outlook**, are **solution-focused**, and view challenges as opportunities for growth. Resilience is not an innate quality but a skill that can be cultivated through practice.

9.6.2 Developing a Growth Mindset

- **Growth vs. Fixed Mindset**: A **growth mindset** involves believing that abilities and qualities can be developed through effort and learning, whereas a **fixed mindset** involves seeing abilities as unchangeable. In weight management, a growth mindset means viewing setbacks as opportunities to learn and improve, rather than as failures.

- **Challenging Limiting Beliefs: Limiting beliefs** are negative thoughts that prevent progress, such as "I can't lose weight" or "I'll always be overweight." Challenging these beliefs by asking, "Is this thought true?" or "What evidence do I have to support this?" can help reframe them in a more positive light. Replacing limiting beliefs with **affirmations** like "I am capable of change" or "Every effort I make is a step forward" fosters a growth mindset.

9.6.3 Learning from Setbacks

Setbacks are an inevitable part of any journey, including weight loss. How you respond to setbacks determines whether you can overcome them and continue moving forward.

- **Analyzing Setbacks Without Judgment**: When experiencing a setback, take time to **analyze** it without self-judgment. Ask yourself, "What led to this situation?" "What can I learn from it?" and "What can I do differently next time?" This reflection helps identify areas for improvement without being overly critical.

- **Using Setbacks as Opportunities for Growth**: Reframing setbacks as opportunities for growth allows you to take a proactive approach to challenges. For example, if emotional eating occurs after a stressful day, consider how to better manage stress in the future—such as through **deep breathing, journaling,** or **reaching out to a friend**.

9.6.4 Practicing Self-Compassion

Self-compassion involves treating yourself with **kindness** and **understanding**, especially during times of struggle or failure. Many individuals who struggle with weight have a tendency to be harshly critical of themselves, but this often leads to feelings of guilt and shame, which can perpetuate unhealthy behaviors.

- **Three Components of Self-Compassion**: According to psychologist **Kristin Neff**, self-compassion has three components:

- o **Self-Kindness**: Being gentle and understanding with yourself, rather than harsh or self-critical.

- o **Common Humanity**: Recognizing that everyone makes mistakes and experiences difficulties; you are not alone.

- o **Mindfulness**: Being present with your feelings without over-identifying with them. Acknowledge negative emotions, but don't let them define you.

- **Self-Compassion Practices**: Practice **self-compassion** by speaking to yourself the way you would speak to a friend. When you experience a setback, ask yourself, "What would I say to a friend in this situation?" Write yourself a **compassionate letter** when you're struggling or repeat affirmations like, "I am doing my best, and that's enough."

9.7 Nurturing a Positive Body Image

9.7.1 Understanding Body Image

Body image is the perception of one's own body and how one feels about their physical appearance. It is influenced by a variety of factors, including **societal ideals, media, family, and peers**. Developing a positive body image is crucial for emotional well-being and sustainable weight management.

- **Negative Body Image**: Negative body image involves dissatisfaction with one's appearance, preoccupation with perceived flaws, and comparison to unrealistic standards. Negative body image is associated with **low self-esteem, depression**, and **disordered eating behaviors.**

- **Positive Body Image**: Positive body image means accepting, appreciating, and respecting your body as it is, regardless of its shape or size. It involves focusing on what your body can do and recognizing your worth beyond physical appearance.

9.7.2 Factors That Influence Body Image

- **Media and Societal Ideals**: Media often portrays a narrow and unrealistic standard of beauty that can impact body image. **Social media**, in particular, contributes to negative body image through **filtered** and **edited** images. Understanding that these images are not realistic representations helps reduce the pressure to conform to these ideals.

- **Family and Peer Influences**: Comments from **family** and **peers** about weight, appearance, or eating habits can also shape body image. **Positive role models** and **supportive family environments** can foster body appreciation, while negative comments can contribute to body dissatisfaction.

- **Comparison: Social comparison** is another significant factor in shaping body image. Constantly comparing oneself to others, especially in terms of weight or appearance, can lead to body dissatisfaction. Recognizing that every individual has a unique body and journey can help reduce the urge to compare.

9.7.3 Strategies for Building a Positive Body Image

- **Practice Body Neutrality: Body neutrality** involves focusing on what the body can do rather than how it looks. It is about appreciating your body for its strength, health, and capabilities, rather than its physical appearance. For example, instead of focusing on whether your legs look a certain way, focus on their ability to carry you through a **run, dance**, or **hike**.

- **Limit Exposure to Negative Influences**: Curate your **social media feed** to include accounts that promote **body positivity, diverse body types**, and **self-acceptance**. Unfollow accounts that make you feel bad about your body or promote unrealistic ideals.

- **Affirmations and Positive Self-Talk**: Use positive affirmations to counter negative thoughts about your body. Affirmations like "My body is strong," "I am grateful for my body," or "I deserve to take up space" can help shift focus from criticism to appreciation.

- **Dress for Comfort and Confidence**: Wearing clothes that make you feel comfortable and confident can have a significant impact on body image. Avoid clothing that feels restrictive or makes you self-conscious. Instead, choose outfits that fit well, are comfortable, and reflect your personal style.

9.8 Changing Your Relationship with Food

9.8.1 Moving Away from Diet Culture

Diet culture is the belief system that equates thinness with health and worthiness. It promotes **restriction, weight loss**, and **body control** as a way to achieve happiness and success. Moving away from diet culture involves challenging these beliefs and embracing a more balanced, sustainable approach to health and weight management.

- **Rejecting the "Good vs. Bad" Food Mentality**: One of the hallmarks of diet culture is labeling foods as **"good"** or **"bad."** This can lead to feelings of guilt when eating certain foods, which may lead to restriction or bingeing. Instead, aim to view food as **neutral**—recognize that all foods can fit into a healthy diet and that balance is key.

- **Focusing on Health, Not Weight**: Health is not solely determined by body weight. It is influenced by a variety of factors, including **mental well-being, physical activity, stress management**, and **balanced nutrition**. Shifting the focus away from weight and toward overall health helps develop a more positive relationship with both food and body.

- **Ditching the Scale**: Constantly weighing oneself can lead to fixation on a number rather than focusing on overall well-being. Consider **ditching the scale** or reducing the frequency of weigh-ins. Instead, monitor progress through **non-scale victories** such as increased energy, improved mood, better sleep, or clothing fitting differently.

9.8.2 Developing Food Freedom

Food freedom is the concept of being able to make food choices without feelings of guilt or fear. It involves allowing yourself to enjoy all foods in moderation and trusting your body to guide you.

- **Allowing All Foods**: Restrictive diets often lead to intense cravings and bingeing once the restriction ends. Instead, allow yourself to enjoy **all types of food**. When no food is off-limits, the urgency to overeat it is reduced. Learning to eat in moderation rather than complete avoidance helps build a balanced relationship with food.

- **Listening to Hunger and Fullness Cues**: Trusting and listening to your body's **hunger** and **fullness** cues is central to food freedom. Avoid eating based on arbitrary rules or schedules; instead, pay attention to your body's natural signals and eat when you're hungry and stop when you're full.

- **Satisfying Cravings Without Guilt**: Cravings are normal, and satisfying them in moderation is part of developing a healthy relationship with food. For example, if you're craving chocolate, have a piece of chocolate and savor it mindfully. When cravings are satisfied without guilt, the cycle of deprivation and bingeing is reduced.

9.8.3 Intuitive Eating as an Approach

Intuitive eating is an approach to eating that encourages individuals to trust their body's signals for hunger, fullness, and satisfaction. It was developed by **Evelyn Tribole** and **Elyse Resch** as an antidote to diet culture and emphasizes a positive relationship with food.

- **The Ten Principles of Intuitive Eating**: The ten principles of intuitive eating include:

  - **Rejecting Diet Mentality**: Letting go of the belief that there is a perfect diet that will lead to happiness and success.

  - **Honoring Your Hunger**: Eating when you are hungry to avoid extreme hunger, which can lead to overeating.

- o **Making Peace with Food**: Giving yourself unconditional permission to eat all foods without guilt.

- o **Challenging the Food Police**: Rejecting thoughts that label foods as "good" or "bad" or criticize your eating choices.

- o **Feeling Your Fullness**: Learning to recognize when you are comfortably full and satisfied.

- o **Discovering Satisfaction**: Eating what you truly want and savoring the experience can lead to greater satisfaction with less food.

- o **Coping with Emotions Without Using Food**: Finding ways to cope with emotions that do not involve eating.

- o **Respecting Your Body**: Accepting your body for what it is, rather than trying to change it to fit societal ideals.

- o **Movement—Feel the Difference**: Focusing on the way movement makes you feel rather than just as a means to burn calories.

- o **Honoring Your Health**: Choosing foods that honor your health and taste good, without rigid rules.

- **The Benefits of Intuitive Eating**: Research shows that intuitive eating is associated with **lower BMI, better psychological health**, and **reduced disordered eating behaviors**. It allows individuals to enjoy food without restriction, promoting long-term health and well-being.

9.9 Conclusion: The Emotional and Behavioral Keys to Weight Management Success

The psychology of eating is a complex, multifaceted aspect of weight management. Understanding the emotional and behavioral components of eating is crucial for developing a healthy, sustainable approach to weight loss. Emotional eating, food addiction, negative body image, and the pressures of diet culture are all challenges that can stand in the way of successful weight management.

By addressing the **emotional triggers** of eating, challenging **negative thoughts**, practicing **mindful eating**, building **resilience**, and nurturing a **positive body image**, individuals can transform their relationship with food and body. The goal is to move away from restriction, guilt, and self-criticism and toward **balance, compassion**, and **self-acceptance**.

Weight management is not just about what you eat; it's about why and how you eat. By focusing on the emotional and behavioral aspects of eating, you can develop the tools necessary to maintain weight loss, enjoy food without guilt, and live a healthier, more fulfilling life.

Chapter 11: Transforming Mindset and Self-Identity for Lasting Health and Happiness

11.1 Understanding Mindset and Its Role in Health

11.1.1 Growth Mindset vs. Fixed Mindset

The concept of **mindset**—how we perceive our abilities and potential—has a profound effect on our approach to health and weight management. **Carol Dweck**, a well-known psychologist, introduced the distinction between a **growth mindset** and a **fixed mindset**, which is crucial to understanding one's journey toward health and well-being.

- **Fixed Mindset**: A fixed mindset is the belief that abilities, intelligence, and characteristics are static and cannot be changed. For those with a fixed mindset, failure is seen as an indicator of personal deficiency. When it comes to health and weight management, a fixed mindset may lead individuals to think, "I've always been overweight, and I'll never be able to change." This perspective often results in a lack of motivation, giving up after setbacks, and an inability to persevere when facing challenges.

- **Growth Mindset**: In contrast, a growth mindset is the belief that abilities and characteristics can be developed through dedication, effort, and learning. Individuals with a growth mindset view setbacks as opportunities for growth and improvement rather than as evidence of personal failure. For weight management, adopting a growth mindset means recognizing that challenges are a part of the journey and that progress is achieved through persistence and learning from experiences. For example, a lapse in diet adherence is seen as a learning opportunity, prompting reflection on what led to the setback and how to approach the situation differently in the future.

- **Benefits of a Growth Mindset for Weight Loss**: A growth mindset helps foster **resilience, self-compassion**, and **determination**. Individuals with a growth mindset are more likely to stick with their health goals because they see challenges as part of the process rather than as obstacles that cannot be overcome. This mindset also promotes **experimentation** with different strategies, helping individuals discover what works best for them and adapt their approach as needed.

11.1.2 Shifting from a Fixed to a Growth Mindset

Transitioning from a **fixed mindset** to a **growth mindset** is essential for those seeking lasting health changes. Making this shift requires conscious effort, reflection, and a willingness to challenge one's beliefs about abilities and potential.

- **Recognize Fixed Mindset Thoughts**: The first step is recognizing when you are having **fixed mindset thoughts**. These may sound like, "I'll never be able to do this," "I'm just not disciplined enough," or "I've failed so many times; I can't change." Identifying these thoughts is crucial to challenging and replacing them.

- **Reframe Negative Thoughts**: Once you recognize a fixed mindset thought, practice reframing it into a **growth-oriented perspective**. For example, if you think, "I'm terrible at exercise," reframe it as, "I'm not comfortable with exercise yet, but I can learn and improve with practice." This shift in language opens the door to growth and possibility rather than keeping you stuck in a belief of incapability.

- **Embrace Challenges as Opportunities**: Embracing challenges rather than avoiding them is another key aspect of developing a growth mindset. For instance, if you face a **weight loss plateau**, instead of becoming discouraged, see it as an opportunity to learn more about your body's needs. Perhaps you need to adjust your **calorie intake, increase physical activity**, or **change up your exercise routine**. Viewing challenges as chances to grow and adapt helps maintain motivation and prevents discouragement.

11.1.3 The Role of Self-Talk in Shaping Mindset

The **internal dialogue** we have with ourselves—our **self-talk**—shapes our mindset, influences how we perceive our abilities, and affects our emotional state. Self-talk can either encourage growth and resilience or create self-doubt and limit our potential.

- **Negative Self-Talk and Its Consequences: Negative self-talk** often stems from a fixed mindset and can be a significant barrier to achieving health goals. Thoughts like, "I'm not good enough," "I'll never change," or "I'm a failure" can erode motivation and lead to feelings of hopelessness. Negative self-talk also creates a cycle of **self-fulfilling prophecy;** believing that you can't change makes it more likely that you'll give up when faced with challenges.

- **The Power of Positive Self-Talk: Positive self-talk** is a powerful tool for cultivating a growth mindset and building resilience. It involves using encouraging, supportive, and realistic statements to build confidence and motivation. Examples of positive self-talk include, "I am capable of making healthy changes," "Every small step I take brings me closer to my goal," and "It's okay to make mistakes; I learn from them and keep going."

- **Practicing Self-Compassion: Self-compassionate self-talk** is a specific form of positive self-talk that involves treating yourself with the same kindness and understanding that you would offer a friend. Instead of criticizing yourself for setbacks, practice saying, "This is difficult, but I am learning and growing," or "Everyone makes mistakes; I can learn from this and do better." Self-compassion helps reduce the **guilt** and **shame** that can arise from setbacks, making it easier to stay motivated and committed to your health goals.

11.2 Redefining Self-Identity for Long-Term Change

11.2.1 The Role of Self-Identity in Behavior Change

Self-identity refers to how we perceive ourselves and the labels we use to define who we are. It encompasses our beliefs about our abilities, characteristics, and roles, and it significantly impacts our behaviors and decision-making. Understanding and redefining self-identity is crucial for achieving lasting health changes.

- **Self-Identity and Weight Loss**: For many individuals, their self-identity is tightly connected to their past experiences with weight and health. Someone might see themselves as "always being overweight," "unathletic," or "someone who just can't lose weight." These identities can create internal barriers that make it challenging to change behaviors. If you view yourself as someone who is inherently unhealthy, you may subconsciously make choices that align with that belief, such as avoiding exercise or eating unhealthy foods.

- **Identity-Based Habits**: Behavior change is most sustainable when it aligns with a change in **self-identity**. Instead of focusing solely on the **outcome** (e.g., losing 20 pounds), focus on becoming the type of person who embodies the habits that lead to that outcome. For example, shift your identity to, "I am someone who takes care of my health," or "I am an active person." When your actions align with your self-identity, they feel more natural and sustainable, leading to long-term success.

- **The Concept of "Acting As If"**: One strategy for changing self-identity is to **"act as if"** you already embody the identity you desire. If you want to be someone who prioritizes health, ask yourself, "What would a healthy person do in this situation?" and then take that action. Over time, these actions reinforce your new identity, and you begin to see yourself as someone who values health and wellness.

11.2.2 Redefining Self-Identity After Weight Loss

For those who have successfully lost weight, redefining self-identity is crucial for maintaining weight loss. Many people continue to see themselves as the "overweight person" they once were, which can lead to **self-sabotage** and difficulty sustaining healthy behaviors.

- **Embracing the New Self**: After losing weight, it's important to fully embrace your new self-identity as a **healthy, active individual**. This may involve letting go of old labels and recognizing the progress you've made. Celebrate your achievements and remind yourself that you are no longer defined by your past.

- **Visualizing the Future Self**: Visualization is a powerful tool for reshaping self-identity. Spend time visualizing yourself as the person you want to be—

healthy, strong, and confident. Imagine how you carry yourself, how you feel, and how you respond to challenges. Visualization helps solidify your new self-identity and makes it easier to embody those behaviors in daily life.

- **Avoiding the "Imposter Syndrome"**: Some individuals who have lost weight may feel like an **imposter** in their new body, as if they haven't truly earned their transformation. This feeling can lead to self-sabotage and a return to old habits. To overcome this, remind yourself of the hard work and dedication that went into your transformation. **Journaling** about your journey, acknowledging the challenges you've overcome, and celebrating your successes can help reinforce your new identity.

11.2.3 Building a Healthy Self-Image

A healthy **self-image** is crucial for maintaining physical and emotional well-being. It involves viewing yourself in a positive light, appreciating your body, and recognizing your worth beyond physical appearance.

- **Body Neutrality and Body Appreciation**: Instead of focusing solely on physical appearance, practice **body neutrality** and **body appreciation**. Body neutrality involves accepting your body as it is without assigning positive or negative value to it. Body appreciation goes a step further by recognizing and valuing what your body can do—its strength, resilience, and ability to support you in daily life. Shifting your focus from how your body looks to what it can do helps foster a positive self-image and reduces the pressure to achieve an unrealistic standard of beauty.

- **Challenging Negative Body Talk**: Negative body talk—criticizing your appearance or comparing yourself to others—can be detrimental to self-image. When you catch yourself engaging in negative body talk, practice **challenging those thoughts** and replacing them with positive affirmations. For example, if you find yourself thinking, "My legs are too big," reframe it as, "My legs are strong and allow me to move freely." By consistently challenging negative thoughts, you can build a healthier and more positive self-image.

- **Developing Self-Worth Beyond Appearance**: It's important to recognize that your **self-worth** is not determined by your physical appearance. Your value comes from who you are as a person—your kindness, your talents, your passions, and your relationships. Developing a strong sense of self-worth that isn't tied to your body helps create a more balanced and positive self-identity.

11.3 The Power of Visualization and Affirmations

11.3.1 Visualization for Health and Success

Visualization is the practice of creating mental images of a desired outcome or future self. It's a powerful tool used by athletes, performers, and successful individuals to help them achieve their goals. When it comes to health and weight management, visualization can help reinforce your goals, motivate you, and strengthen your belief in your ability to succeed.

- **How Visualization Works**: The brain has difficulty distinguishing between real and vividly imagined experiences. When you visualize yourself successfully achieving your health goals—whether it's reaching a certain fitness level, maintaining a balanced diet, or feeling confident in your body—your brain creates new neural pathways that reinforce these behaviors, making them feel more achievable and natural.

- **Daily Visualization Practice**: To incorporate visualization into your daily routine, set aside a few minutes each day to close your eyes and **imagine** your future self. Picture yourself engaging in healthy behaviors, such as **exercising, preparing nutritious meals,** or **feeling energized** and confident. Focus on the **sensations, emotions,** and **details** of the experience. The more vividly you can visualize yourself achieving your goals, the more real and attainable they will feel.

- **Visualizing Overcoming Challenges**: In addition to visualizing success, it's also helpful to visualize yourself overcoming challenges. Imagine a situation that might be difficult—such as attending a social event with tempting foods—and picture yourself navigating it successfully. Visualization helps you mentally rehearse positive behaviors, making it more likely that you'll respond in a healthy way when faced with real-life challenges.

11.3.2 Using Affirmations to Reinforce Positive Beliefs

Affirmations are positive statements that reinforce your beliefs about yourself and your abilities. They help counteract negative self-talk and build confidence, motivation, and resilience.

- **Creating Effective Affirmations**: Effective affirmations are **positive, specific**, and **present-focused**. Instead of saying, "I will be healthy," reframe it to, "I am becoming healthier every day by making choices that support my well-being." The present focus helps your brain internalize the statement as true, even if you are still on the journey to becoming healthier.

- **Daily Affirmation Practice**: Incorporate affirmations into your daily routine by repeating them aloud, writing them in a journal, or posting them in visible places like your bathroom mirror or refrigerator. Examples of health-focused affirmations include:

o   "I am capable of making positive changes for my health."

o   "I am worthy of love and care, exactly as I am."

o   "I have the strength and determination to reach my goals."

o   "Every choice I make supports my well-being."

- **The Science Behind Affirmations**: Research shows that affirmations help **reduce stress, improve confidence**, and **promote goal achievement** by activating the brain's reward centers. When you repeat affirmations, you are reinforcing positive beliefs and challenging limiting thoughts, which makes it easier to adopt behaviors that align with your health goals.

11.4 Cultivating Resilience and Emotional Strength

11.4.1 The Importance of Resilience in Health and Weight Maintenance

Resilience is the ability to **bounce back** from setbacks, challenges, or adversity. It is an essential quality for achieving and maintaining health goals because the journey to health is often filled with ups and downs. Developing resilience helps you navigate these challenges without losing motivation or giving up.

- **Setbacks as Opportunities for Growth**: Resilient individuals view setbacks not as failures but as opportunities for growth and learning. When faced with a setback, such as overeating or missing a workout, practice **reflecting** on what led to the setback and what can be done differently next time. This approach helps you learn from your experiences and make adjustments that lead to success.

- **Cultivating a Positive Outlook**: A **positive outlook** is a key component of resilience. It doesn't mean ignoring challenges or pretending that everything is perfect, but rather choosing to focus on the positives and look for solutions. When faced with a challenge, ask yourself, "What can I do about this?" or "What lesson can I learn from this?" Cultivating a positive outlook helps you stay motivated and proactive.

- **Building Coping Mechanisms**: Developing healthy **coping mechanisms** is crucial for resilience. Life is filled with stressors, and how you respond to them impacts your health journey. Instead of turning to food as a way to cope with stress or emotions, develop a toolkit of healthy coping mechanisms, such as **deep breathing, exercise, journaling**, or **talking to a friend**. Having these tools at your disposal helps you respond to stress in a way that supports your well-being.

11.4.2 Embracing Flexibility and Adaptability

Flexibility and **adaptability** are important qualities for long-term success. Life is unpredictable, and the ability to adapt your health habits to different circumstances helps you maintain balance.

- **Letting Go of Perfectionism**: One of the biggest barriers to long-term success is **perfectionism**—the belief that you must follow your health plan perfectly in order to succeed. Perfectionism often leads to an all-or-nothing mentality, where any deviation from the plan is seen as a failure. To cultivate resilience, it's important to let go of perfectionism and embrace **flexibility**. Understand that it's normal to have days when you don't eat perfectly or miss a workout, and that these moments are not failures but part of the process.

- **Adjusting Habits to Fit Different Circumstances**: Life changes—whether it's a new job, moving to a new city, or becoming a parent—often require adjustments to your health habits. Instead of feeling discouraged by these changes, practice **adapting** your habits to fit your new circumstances. For example, if your work schedule changes, find a new time to exercise that works with your current routine. Adaptability helps you maintain consistency, even when your environment changes.

11.5 The Practice of Self-Love and Acceptance

11.5.1 Understanding Self-Love and Its Impact on Health

Self-love is the practice of accepting and caring for yourself as you are, without conditions. It involves recognizing your worth, treating yourself with kindness, and making choices that support your well-being. Self-love is a foundational component of a successful health journey because it influences how you treat yourself and the choices you make for your health.

- **Self-Love vs. Self-Criticism**: Many individuals are harshly self-critical, believing that being tough on themselves is necessary for success. However, self-criticism often leads to feelings of **shame, guilt**, and **unworthiness**, which can undermine motivation and lead to self-sabotaging behaviors. In contrast, self-love involves treating yourself with the same kindness and compassion you would offer a loved one. It means encouraging yourself, being patient, and recognizing that you are deserving of care, regardless of your weight or appearance.

- **Making Choices from a Place of Love**: When you love yourself, you make choices that support your well-being—not because you feel obligated to or because you're trying to meet someone else's standards, but because you genuinely care for yourself. This means choosing **nourishing foods**, engaging in **physical activity** that you enjoy, getting **adequate rest**, and setting **healthy boundaries**. Self-love creates a positive foundation for long-term health and happiness.

11.5.2 Practicing Self-Acceptance

Self-acceptance is the practice of accepting all aspects of yourself—both the positive and the less desirable—without judgment. It means recognizing that you are inherently worthy, regardless of your body size, shape, or the number on the scale.

- **Accepting the Present While Aiming for Change**: Self-acceptance does not mean complacency or giving up on self-improvement. Rather, it means accepting yourself as you are in the present moment while still striving for positive change. It's possible to want to improve your health while also appreciating where you are now. By accepting yourself, you create a supportive internal environment that fosters growth and change.

- **Overcoming the "If-Then" Trap**: Many individuals fall into the "**if-then**" trap—believing that they will only be worthy of love or acceptance if they achieve a certain weight or appearance. This mindset creates a constant state of dissatisfaction and prevents true happiness. Instead of basing your self-worth on external achievements, practice accepting yourself as you are. Recognize that your value does not depend on your weight, and that you are worthy of love and acceptance right now.

11.6 The Process of Growth Beyond Weight Loss

11.6.1 Setting New Goals for Personal Growth

After achieving weight loss, it's important to continue setting new goals that foster personal growth and fulfillment. While weight loss may have been your initial goal, there is much more to health and happiness than a number on the scale.

- **Health and Fitness Goals**: After reaching your weight loss goal, consider setting **health and fitness goals** that focus on building strength, improving endurance, or mastering a new skill. Examples include running a **5k**, taking up **yoga**, learning to **dance**, or improving your **flexibility**. Setting new goals helps you stay engaged and motivated while continuing to improve your overall health.

- **Emotional and Mental Well-Being**: Personal growth extends beyond physical health. Setting goals related to **emotional and mental well-being** helps create a balanced and fulfilling life. This could involve practicing **mindfulness**, working on **stress management**, or exploring **therapy** to improve emotional health. Focusing on emotional and mental growth ensures that you continue to evolve and thrive.

- **Learning and Growth Opportunities**: Embrace opportunities for learning and growth outside of weight management. Take up a new **hobby, learn a new language**, pursue a **career goal**, or engage in **creative projects**. Growth in other areas of life contributes to overall happiness and well-being and helps create a fulfilling and meaningful life beyond weight loss.

11.6.2 Becoming a Source of Inspiration

Your journey of weight loss and health transformation has the potential to inspire others. Sharing your experiences, challenges, and successes can motivate and encourage others to pursue their own health goals.

- **Leading by Example**: One of the most powerful ways to inspire others is by **leading by example**. Live in a way that embodies health, self-love, and positivity. When others see you making healthy choices, practicing resilience, and embracing self-acceptance, they are more likely to feel empowered to do the same.

- **Sharing Your Story**: Consider sharing your story with others, whether through **social media**, **blogging**, or **community groups**. Your story may help someone else who is struggling, showing them that change is possible and providing them with valuable insights from your experience. Sharing your story also helps reinforce your own growth and transformation, reminding you of how far you've come.

- **Supporting Others on Their Journey**: Offer support and encouragement to others who are on their own health journey. Whether it's a friend, family member, or coworker, being a source of support helps you stay connected to your own values and goals. It also reinforces the idea that health is a lifelong journey, and we all benefit from support and encouragement along the way.

Chapter 12: The Social and Cultural Dynamics of Weight Loss and Health

12.1 The Impact of Social Relationships on Weight Management

12.1.1 The Role of Social Support in Health Success

Social support is a crucial factor in achieving and maintaining weight loss and overall health. It provides

motivation, **accountability**, and **emotional encouragement** throughout the weight management journey. Relationships with friends, family, coworkers, and support groups can either positively or negatively influence health behaviors.

- **Types of Social Support**: Social support can be categorized into different types:

  - **Emotional Support**: This involves empathy, care, encouragement, and reassurance. Emotional support helps individuals feel understood and motivated, particularly during challenging times. Having someone say, "I'm proud of you," or "You're doing great, keep going," can provide much-needed confidence and motivation.

  - **Informational Support: Informational support** involves providing guidance, advice, and information to help individuals make informed health decisions. It could come from friends sharing recipes, family members suggesting exercise routines, or support groups providing helpful resources.

  - **Practical Support**: This type of support includes practical help, such as preparing healthy meals, going to the gym together, or helping with grocery shopping. **Practical support** reduces barriers to making healthy choices and ensures that individuals have what they need to succeed.

- **The Importance of Accountability: Accountability** is a key aspect of social support that can enhance motivation and adherence to health behaviors. Whether it's a workout buddy who ensures you exercise regularly or a friend you check in with about your eating habits, accountability provides structure and helps keep you on track. Knowing that someone else is aware of your goals and progress can be a powerful motivator.

- **Choosing Supportive Relationships**: Surrounding yourself with people who understand and respect your health goals is essential for success. Supportive relationships are those in which individuals are not only encouraging but also nonjudgmental. People who respect your choices and offer encouragement without criticism create a positive environment that fosters long-term behavior change. If certain relationships are not supportive of your health goals, setting boundaries or limiting exposure to those individuals may be necessary to protect your progress.

12.1.2 Navigating Challenging Social Relationships

Not all social relationships are supportive. Sometimes, well-meaning friends or family members can unintentionally hinder your progress, either by encouraging you to eat unhealthy foods or by expressing skepticism about your health goals.

- **Managing Food Pushers: Food pushers** are individuals who encourage you to eat more or eat foods that do not align with your health goals. They may do this out of love, tradition, or simply not understanding your goals. To manage food pushers, it's helpful to be polite but assertive. Practice phrases like, "Thank you, but I'm trying to make healthier choices right now," or "It looks delicious, but I'm not hungry." Setting boundaries helps ensure that you stay in control of your choices without offending others.

- **Addressing Skepticism**: Some friends or family members may express skepticism about your health journey, either by doubting your ability to succeed or questioning the value of your goals. Skepticism can be discouraging and may undermine your confidence. To address this, communicate your goals clearly and emphasize why they are important to you. You can say, "I know this is important for my health, and I feel better when I make these choices." It's also helpful to remind yourself that your goals are valid, regardless of others' opinions.

- **Dealing with Negative Influence**: There may be individuals in your life who are actively unsupportive or even sabotage your efforts—whether intentionally or unintentionally. These relationships can be challenging to navigate, especially if they involve close family members or friends. In such cases, setting clear boundaries and limiting exposure may be necessary. Surrounding yourself with supportive people—whether in person or through online communities—can help counterbalance negative influences.

12.1.3 Building a Health-Focused Social Network

Creating a **health-focused social network** involves surrounding yourself with people who share your values and goals related to health and well-being. This network can be made up of friends, family, coworkers, or members of community groups who are also focused on leading a healthy lifestyle.

- **Connecting with Like-Minded Individuals**: Finding like-minded individuals who share your health goals helps create a sense of community and support. This could involve joining **fitness classes, online support groups**, or **local wellness communities**. Connecting with others who are on a similar journey provides opportunities for shared activities, mutual encouragement, and learning from one another.

- **Fitness and Wellness Communities: Fitness communities**, such as running clubs, yoga studios, or group fitness classes, provide a sense of accountability and camaraderie. Participating in group activities creates motivation through the shared experience of working toward similar goals. Similarly, **wellness communities**, such as **nutrition workshops** or **mindfulness groups**, provide educational support and foster a sense of community.

- **Finding an Accountability Partner**: An **accountability partner** is someone who shares your health goals and is committed to helping you stay on track. Whether it's a friend, family member, or coworker, having someone to check in with regularly provides motivation and consistency. You can share your progress, celebrate successes, and discuss challenges together. This mutual support helps keep both of you engaged in your health journey.

12.2 Family Dynamics and Cultural Influences on Weight Management

12.2.1 The Role of Family in Shaping Eating Habits

Family dynamics play a significant role in shaping **eating habits**, especially during childhood and adolescence. The attitudes, beliefs, and behaviors of family members often influence how individuals view food, exercise, and health.

- **Family as a Source of Habits**: Eating habits are often established in childhood, based on the types of foods that are available and the attitudes of family members toward food. If a family has a habit of eating **high-calorie, processed foods**, children are likely to adopt similar habits. Conversely, families that prioritize **home-cooked meals** and **balanced nutrition** tend to raise individuals with a positive relationship with food.

- **Family Meals and Their Impact: Family meals** can have a positive impact on health. Eating together provides an opportunity to model healthy eating behaviors, create balanced meals, and foster a positive relationship with food. Research suggests that individuals who regularly eat meals with their family are more likely to consume **fruits, vegetables,** and **whole grains** and are less likely to engage in unhealthy eating behaviors.

- **Overcoming Unhealthy Family Dynamics**: For some individuals, family dynamics may include unhealthy habits, such as frequent consumption of **fast food**, **overeating**, or a lack of **physical activity**. Overcoming these dynamics requires setting personal boundaries and developing new habits that align with your health goals. For example, if your family frequently orders **takeout**, offer to cook a **healthy meal** that everyone can enjoy together. It's also important to communicate your goals openly and let family members know how they can support you.

12.2.2 Cultural Norms and Their Impact on Weight and Health

Cultural norms shape beliefs about **body image, health, and food**, which can influence weight management behaviors. Culture can either support or hinder health goals, depending on the values and traditions that are emphasized.

- **Cultural Attitudes Toward Body Image**: Different cultures have varying ideals of what constitutes a healthy or attractive body. In some cultures, **thinness** is highly valued and equated with health and success, leading to pressure to conform to unrealistic standards. In other cultures, **larger body sizes** may be associated with health, fertility, or prosperity. Understanding how cultural attitudes influence your perception of your body can help you develop a more balanced and realistic view of health.

- **Food Traditions and Dietary Habits**: Food is an important part of cultural identity, and traditional foods are often rich in **flavor, calories**, and **symbolic meaning**. While cultural foods can be nutritious, some traditional dishes may be high in **fats, sugars**, or **refined carbohydrates**. Navigating cultural food traditions while maintaining health goals can be challenging, but it is possible to make healthier adaptations to traditional dishes without losing their cultural significance. For example, consider **baking** instead of **frying** or using **healthier fats** in traditional recipes.

- **The Role of Celebrations**: Cultural celebrations and holidays are often centered around food, which can make maintaining health goals challenging. Instead of avoiding celebrations, focus on **moderation** and **mindful indulgence**. Allow yourself to enjoy cultural foods, but be mindful of portion sizes and choose healthier options when possible. Celebrating the cultural aspects of an event—such as spending time with loved ones, engaging in traditional activities, or focusing on the meaning behind the celebration—can also help shift the emphasis away from food.

12.2.3 Balancing Cultural Identity with Health Goals

Maintaining a healthy lifestyle while honoring cultural identity can be challenging, but it is possible to achieve balance by making conscious choices and practicing **moderation.**

- **Modifying Traditional Recipes**: One way to balance cultural identity with health goals is to modify traditional recipes to make them healthier. This might include using **leaner proteins, reducing added sugars,** or **increasing vegetables.** Small changes can make a big difference in the overall nutritional profile of a dish while still preserving its cultural significance and flavor.

- **Fostering Cultural Pride Without Guilt**: It's important to foster a sense of **cultural pride** without guilt. Cultural foods and traditions are an essential part of identity, and feeling guilty about enjoying them can create a negative relationship with food. Instead, practice enjoying cultural foods mindfully and in moderation, without feelings of guilt or deprivation. Recognize that your cultural identity is an important part of who you are and that it's possible to honor it while still pursuing health goals.

- **Connecting with Culturally Aligned Health Communities**: For individuals who feel that their cultural background is not well-represented in mainstream health communities, finding **culturally aligned health communities** can be beneficial. These communities provide support, understanding, and guidance that is tailored to your unique cultural context. Whether it's a **cooking class** focused on healthier versions of traditional dishes, a **fitness group** for people of similar backgrounds, or an **online community** that celebrates cultural diversity in health, connecting with like-minded individuals helps create a sense of belonging and support.

12.3 Media Influence and Societal Pressures

12.3.1 The Role of Media in Shaping Body Image

The media has a significant influence on how individuals perceive **body image** and **health**. Images, advertisements, social media, and even movies and TV shows create and reinforce cultural standards of beauty and health, which can affect self-esteem and motivation.

- **The Pressure of Unrealistic Standards**: Media often portrays an **idealized version of beauty**, characterized by **thinness, muscularity**, or specific body proportions. These ideals are often unattainable for most individuals and do not reflect the natural diversity of body shapes and sizes. Constant exposure to these unrealistic standards can lead to **body dissatisfaction, negative self-image**, and **unhealthy behaviors** in an attempt to conform to these ideals.

- **Social Media and Its Impact: Social media** has become a powerful tool for shaping body image, with platforms like **Instagram, TikTok**, and **Facebook** presenting curated and edited versions of people's lives. Influencers and celebrities often promote **diets, weight loss supplements**, and **fitness routines**, contributing to the pressure to look a certain way. The use of filters and photo-editing tools creates an unrealistic perception of beauty, leading to comparison and dissatisfaction. It's important to remember that social media often presents a highlight reel, not the full reality.

- **The Role of Advertising: Advertising** also plays a role in shaping body image and health behaviors. Products that promise **weight loss, anti-aging**, or **body sculpting** are often marketed in a way that suggests that physical appearance is the key to happiness and success. Recognizing the persuasive tactics used in advertising can help you make more informed choices and resist the pressure to buy into unrealistic ideals.

12.3.2 Strategies for Cultivating a Positive Media Environment

While it's difficult to avoid media influence entirely, there are strategies you can use to cultivate a **positive media environment** that supports a healthy body image and well-being.

- **Curate Your Social Media Feed**: Take control of what you see by curating your social media feed. Unfollow accounts that make you feel negative about yourself or that promote unrealistic standards of beauty. Instead, follow accounts that promote **body positivity, diversity, health**, and **self-acceptance**. This can help shift your focus from comparison to inspiration and encourage a more positive outlook on health.

- **Limit Media Exposure**: If you find that certain forms of media negatively affect your self-esteem or motivation, consider limiting your exposure to them. This might mean reducing the time spent on social media, avoiding certain TV shows, or being mindful of the advertisements you consume. Being intentional about your media consumption helps reduce its impact on your self-perception.

- **Seek Out Positive Role Models**: Look for **positive role models** who promote a balanced and realistic approach to health and well-being. This might include **athletes, activists, health professionals**, or **influencers** who focus on **strength, health**, and **confidence** rather than appearance. Surrounding yourself with positive influences helps shift your focus from unrealistic ideals to achievable and meaningful health goals.

12.3.3 Building Resilience Against Societal Pressures

Societal pressures regarding **body image, weight**, and **appearance** can be challenging to navigate. Building resilience against these pressures helps maintain focus on your health goals without being swayed by external expectations.

- **Questioning Societal Norms**: Developing resilience involves questioning **societal norms** and recognizing that beauty and health are not one-size-fits-all. Ask yourself whether the standards you are striving for are realistic or if they have been imposed by media, advertising, or cultural expectations. Challenge the notion that **thinness** equates to **health** or that **muscularity** equates to **strength**. Remind yourself that health looks different for everyone and that your value is not determined by your appearance.

- **Developing Internal Validation**: Rather than seeking validation from external sources—such as social media likes, comments, or compliments—focus on developing **internal validation**. Internal validation comes from within and involves recognizing your own worth and celebrating your achievements without needing external approval. Practicing **gratitude, self-reflection**, and **positive affirmations** helps reinforce internal validation and reduces the need for societal approval.

- **Celebrating Body Diversity**: Celebrating and appreciating **body diversity** helps counteract the narrow standards promoted by society. Recognize that bodies come in all shapes and sizes, and that health cannot be determined by appearance alone. Celebrate the unique qualities of your own body and appreciate what it allows you to do. By embracing diversity, you create a positive and inclusive mindset that supports both your health journey and the well-being of others.

12.4 The Effect of Social Comparison and Peer Influence

12.4.1 Social Comparison and Its Impact on Health Behaviors

- **The Influence of Social Circles**: Your **social circle**—friends, coworkers, and acquaintances—can significantly impact your health behaviors through both direct influence and subconscious comparison. For instance, if your friends engage in regular physical activity, you may feel more motivated to exercise as well. On the other hand, if your social group often indulges in unhealthy behaviors, such as **overeating** or **drinking alcohol excessively**, you may feel pressured to join in to fit in.

- **Social Media and Comparison: Social media** amplifies social comparison, as people often post their best moments—workouts, healthy meals, weight loss achievements—creating a curated version of their lives. Constant exposure to these idealized images can lead to feelings of **inadequacy** and **self-doubt**, making it difficult to maintain motivation for your own health journey. Recognizing that social media often showcases the highlights rather than the whole picture can help reduce the negative impact of comparison.

- **Healthy vs. Unhealthy Comparisons**: The impact of social comparison on your health largely depends on how you use it. **Healthy comparisons** can provide inspiration and motivate positive behavior changes. For example, seeing a friend succeed in a fitness goal might encourage you to set a similar goal. However, **unhealthy comparisons**—such as constantly comparing your progress to others or feeling inferior—can lead to **demotivation** and **self-sabotage**. It's important to focus on your own journey and understand that everyone's health path is unique.

12.4.2 Strategies for Minimizing Negative Social Comparison

Reducing the impact of negative social comparison is key to maintaining a positive outlook on your health journey. Here are some strategies for minimizing its effects:

- **Focus on Your Personal Growth**: One way to minimize negative social comparison is to focus on your **personal growth** and celebrate your own achievements, no matter how small. Tracking your **progress over time**—such as improvements in **strength, endurance, flexibility**, or **eating habits**—helps you recognize your efforts and value the progress you've made, rather than comparing yourself to others.

- **Use Others as Inspiration, Not a Benchmark**: Rather than comparing your progress to someone else's, use their journey as **inspiration** for what is possible. For example, if a friend has successfully adopted a healthy eating routine or achieved a fitness goal, let it inspire you to work towards your own goals without feeling inferior or discouraged. Recognize that everyone starts from a different place and has their own unique challenges.

- **Limit Exposure to Triggering Content**: If social media or certain individuals trigger feelings of inadequacy, consider limiting your exposure to them. Curate your **social media feed** to include accounts that promote **body positivity**, **self-acceptance**, and **health diversity**, and unfollow accounts that lead to **negative feelings** or pressure to conform to unrealistic standards.

- **Practice Gratitude for Your Body**: Practicing **gratitude** for what your body can do helps counteract negative comparisons. Instead of focusing on what you perceive as flaws or areas for improvement, take time each day to appreciate your body's capabilities—whether it's walking, dancing, hugging a loved one, or simply functioning day-to-day. Shifting your focus to appreciation helps foster a positive relationship with your body.

12.4.3 Peer Influence and Behavioral Mimicry

Peer influence plays a significant role in shaping behaviors, especially when it comes to health-related habits like **diet**, **exercise**, and **sleep**. The tendency to adopt behaviors similar to those of your peers—often referred to as **behavioral mimicry**—is a natural part of social dynamics and can be either helpful or harmful, depending on the habits being modeled.

- **Positive Peer Influence**: When surrounded by peers who prioritize **healthy eating**, **regular exercise**, and **self-care**, you are more likely to adopt similar habits. Positive peer influence encourages accountability, shared activities, and the opportunity to learn from others' experiences. For example, joining a **running club** or **workout group** provides both motivation and a supportive environment that makes sticking to fitness goals easier.

- **Negative Peer Influence**: On the other hand, peers who engage in **unhealthy behaviors**, such as **overeating, excessive drinking**, or avoiding physical activity, can negatively influence your health journey. In such situations, it's important to establish boundaries, communicate your goals, and, if necessary, limit exposure to individuals whose habits are not aligned with your goals.

- **Setting Boundaries and Leading by Example**: When dealing with peer influence that doesn't align with your health goals, it's important to set clear boundaries. For example, if your friends frequently suggest **unhealthy restaurants**, offer alternatives that fit your goals, such as suggesting a restaurant with healthier options. By standing firm in your decisions and leading by example, you not only protect your own progress but also influence others to make healthier choices.

12.5 Creating a Positive Social Environment for Health Success

12.5.1 Engaging in Community and Group Activities

Engaging in **community and group activities** helps create a sense of belonging and provides a supportive environment for maintaining health and wellness. Being part of a community with shared interests in health, fitness, or well-being fosters **motivation, accountability, and encouragement.**

- **Joining Fitness Classes or Clubs**: Participating in **fitness classes** or joining **sports clubs** creates a sense of community and accountability. Whether it's a **yoga studio, cycling class**, or **hiking group**, shared activities make physical activity more enjoyable and provide an opportunity to connect with others who share similar health goals.

- **Community Events and Wellness Programs**: Many communities offer **wellness programs** and events, such as **nutrition workshops, walking groups**, or **health fairs**. Engaging in these activities helps you stay informed, build new skills, and connect with like-minded individuals who are also committed to improving their health.

- **Online Health Communities**: In addition to in-person communities, **online health communities** provide support, information, and motivation for individuals pursuing health goals. Joining online forums, **social media groups**, or **virtual fitness challenges** can help you stay connected to others on a similar journey, even if you don't have a strong in-person support network.

12.5.2 Strengthening Relationships That Support Health Goals

The quality of your relationships plays a significant role in maintaining long-term health. Strengthening relationships that support your health goals helps create a positive social environment that fosters both **physical** and **emotional well-being**.

- **Communicating Needs and Boundaries**: Communication is key to creating supportive relationships. Let your friends and family know about your health goals and what kind of support you need. For example, if you're trying to eat healthier, ask your partner to support your decision by cooking meals together or avoiding bringing unhealthy snacks into the house. Setting clear **boundaries** and **expressing your needs** helps those around you understand how they can support you.

- **Prioritizing Relationships That Add Value**: Focus on nurturing relationships that uplift and support you. These are the relationships that provide **encouragement**, **understanding**, and **emotional support** during your health journey. Spending time with people who value your well-being and celebrate your progress—no matter how small—makes it easier to stay motivated and committed to your goals.

- **Encouraging Mutual Support**: Mutual support involves not only receiving support from others but also offering support in return. When you help others achieve their health goals—whether by encouraging a friend to exercise, preparing a healthy meal for a loved one, or simply listening to someone's challenges—you reinforce your own commitment to health. This shared support strengthens relationships and creates a sense of community that benefits everyone involved.

12.5.3 Creating a Health-Friendly Home Environment

Your **home environment** plays a crucial role in maintaining health and well-being. Creating a home environment that supports healthy behaviors makes it easier to make positive choices consistently.

- **Stocking Nutritious Foods**: The foods that are available in your home are the ones you are most likely to eat. Stocking your kitchen with **fruits, vegetables, whole grains, lean proteins**, and **healthy snacks** ensures that nutritious options are readily available. Limiting the availability of **processed, high-calorie foods** helps reduce temptation and makes it easier to maintain healthy eating habits.

- **Establishing Spaces for Physical Activity**: Create spaces in your home where you can comfortably engage in **physical activity**. This doesn't require an entire home gym—even a small area for **yoga, stretching**, or using **resistance bands** can help you stay active. Having a dedicated space for exercise serves as a reminder of your health goals and makes it more convenient to fit movement into your daily routine.

- **Cultivating a Positive Emotional Environment**: The emotional environment of your home is just as important as the physical one. Creating a space that feels **calm, positive,** and **supportive** helps reduce stress and fosters well-being. This might involve setting up a **meditation area,** decorating your space with **inspirational quotes,** or practicing **gratitude** as a family. Cultivating a positive emotional environment helps support both mental and physical health.

12.6 Building Community Support Systems for Health Equity

12.6.1 Understanding Health Inequities

Health inequities are differences in health outcomes that are avoidable and unfair, often resulting from social, economic, and environmental factors. These inequities can affect access to **healthy foods, safe environments for exercise,** and **healthcare,** making it more challenging for some individuals to achieve and maintain health.

- **Access to Healthy Foods**: In many communities, especially **low-income areas,** access to **affordable, nutritious foods** is limited. These areas, often referred to as **food deserts,** lack grocery stores that offer fresh produce, whole grains, and lean proteins, while **convenience stores** and **fast food** options are more readily available. This disparity makes it challenging for individuals in these communities to maintain a healthy diet.

- **Safe Environments for Physical Activity**: Access to **safe environments** for physical activity is another factor that contributes to health inequities. In some communities, lack of **parks, recreation centers,** or **safe sidewalks** makes it difficult for individuals to engage in physical activity. Safety concerns, such as crime or poor lighting, may also discourage people from walking, running, or exercising outdoors.

- **Barriers to Healthcare:** Access to **healthcare** and **preventive services** is essential for maintaining health, but many individuals face barriers, such as lack of **health insurance, high costs,** or **limited availability** of providers. These barriers can prevent individuals from receiving necessary screenings, treatments, or support for health management, exacerbating health inequities.

12.6.2 Advocating for Health Equity in Your Community

Addressing health inequities requires collective action and advocacy. By getting involved in your community and advocating for policies and programs that promote **health equity,** you can help create an environment where everyone has the opportunity to live a healthy life.

- **Supporting Community Initiatives:** Many communities have initiatives aimed at improving access to **healthy foods, safe recreational spaces,** and **health services.** Supporting these initiatives—whether through **volunteering, donations,** or **advocacy**—helps create positive change. This might include supporting local **farmers' markets,** participating in community clean-up events to improve local parks, or advocating for new **bike lanes** or **walking paths**.

- **Advocating for Policy Change: Policy change** is a powerful tool for addressing health inequities. Advocating for policies that promote **access to healthy foods, affordable healthcare**, and **safe environments** for physical activity can help create systemic change. This might involve **contacting local representatives**, attending **community meetings**, or joining organizations that work toward **public health** and **health equity**.

- **Educating and Empowering Others: Education** is a key factor in promoting health equity. By educating others in your community about **nutrition, exercise,** and **self-care**, you can help empower them to make informed choices about their health. Hosting **workshops, sharing resources**, or simply having conversations about health and wellness helps spread knowledge and support within the community.

12.6.3 Building Inclusive Health Communities

Building **inclusive health communities** involves creating spaces where individuals from all backgrounds feel welcome, supported, and empowered to pursue health and well-being.

- **Promoting Cultural Competence: Cultural competence** is the ability to understand, respect, and address the diverse cultural backgrounds and health beliefs of individuals within a community.

Promoting cultural competence within health communities helps ensure that everyone feels understood and respected. This might involve **offering multilingual resources**, respecting **cultural dietary practices**, or incorporating **culturally relevant activities** into wellness programs.

- **Ensuring Accessibility:** Ensuring that health resources are **accessible** to everyone is an important aspect of building inclusive communities. This includes providing **physical accessibility** for individuals with disabilities, offering **financial assistance** for low-income individuals, and creating **safe spaces** where people feel comfortable participating in health activities.

- **Creating Safe and Supportive Spaces**: Creating **safe and supportive spaces** is crucial for fostering community health. This means ensuring that health communities are **nonjudgmental, inclusive**, and **encouraging**. Everyone, regardless of their starting point, should feel welcome and supported in pursuing their health goals. A sense of belonging and community support helps individuals stay motivated and committed to their well-being.

Chapter 13: The Science of Sustainable Habits: Building a Lifestyle That Lasts

13.1 Understanding Habit Formation: The Basics

13.1.1 What Are Habits and Why Are They Important?

Habits are automatic behaviors that we perform without conscious thought. They are formed through repetition and become part of our daily routine, helping us conserve mental energy. Habits play a crucial role in health and weight management because they allow us to make consistent, positive choices without needing to rely solely on willpower or motivation.

- **The Role of Habits in Health**: Health behaviors such as **eating nutritious foods, exercising regularly, staying hydrated**, and **getting enough sleep** are most sustainable when they become habits. When these behaviors are automatic, they require less effort and become a natural part of daily life. In contrast, when health behaviors require constant conscious effort, they are more difficult to maintain over the long term.

- **The Habit Loop: Charles Duhigg**, in his book **"The Power of Habit"**, describes the concept of the **habit loop**, which consists of three parts: **cue, routine**, and **reward**. The cue is the trigger that initiates the habit, the routine is the behavior itself, and the reward is the positive outcome that reinforces the habit. Understanding this loop helps you create new habits and modify existing ones.

- **Automaticity and Cognitive Load**: One of the reasons habits are powerful is because they reduce **cognitive load**—the amount of mental effort required to perform a behavior. By making health behaviors automatic, you free up mental energy for other tasks. For example, if going for a morning walk is a habit, you don't need to think about it or muster motivation; it's simply part of your routine.

13.1 Understanding Habit Formation: The Basics (continued)

13.1.2 The Process of Habit Formation (continued)

- **Using Triggers to Initiate Habits**: A **trigger** (or cue) is an event or a prompt that initiates a behavior. Triggers can be **external** (such as an alarm clock or a specific time of day) or **internal** (such as a feeling of stress or boredom). To build a sustainable habit, it's helpful to establish consistent triggers. For example, if you want to start meditating daily, use a specific time of day (such as right after waking up) as your trigger. Triggers help create a reliable context that cues the behavior, making it easier to remember and perform.

- **Environment as a Trigger**: Your **environment** plays a key role in habit formation, as the cues around you can prompt certain behaviors. Designing your environment to support healthy habits—such as placing a **water bottle** on your desk to remind you to drink water or leaving your **workout clothes** out the night before—creates visual triggers that prompt desired actions. On the flip side, removing triggers for unhealthy behaviors (e.g., keeping **junk food** out of sight) can reduce the likelihood of engaging in those behaviors.

- **Building Habit Stacks: Habit stacking** is a technique that involves linking a new habit to an existing one, making it easier to remember. For example, if you already brush your teeth every morning, you could "stack" a new habit onto that routine, such as doing **five minutes of stretching** right afterward. By anchoring the new habit to an established one, you take advantage of an existing routine, making the formation of the new habit more seamless.

13.1.3 Reward Systems and Reinforcement

Rewards are an essential part of the habit loop, as they provide positive reinforcement that encourages the repetition of a behavior. The reward doesn't have to be significant; it just needs to provide a sense of satisfaction that makes you want to repeat the behavior.

- **Immediate Rewards**: The key to reinforcing a new habit is to ensure that there is some form of **immediate reward** following the behavior. For instance, the **endorphin rush** after a workout, the feeling of relaxation after meditating, or the sense of accomplishment after completing a task can all serve as immediate rewards. These positive feelings help cement the behavior as something enjoyable or satisfying.

- **Intrinsic vs. Extrinsic Rewards**: Rewards can be **intrinsic** (internal) or **extrinsic** (external). **Intrinsic rewards** include feelings of pride, accomplishment, or well-being. These types of rewards are the most powerful for building long-term habits, as they are inherently linked to the behavior itself. **Extrinsic rewards**, such as treating yourself to a new book or a favorite snack after reaching a milestone, can also be helpful, particularly in the early stages of habit formation. However, it's important to eventually transition to intrinsic rewards for lasting habit change.

- **Celebration as a Reinforcement: Celebrating** small wins is another way to reinforce new habits. Taking a moment to acknowledge your efforts and feel proud of your progress—even if it's something small—helps release **dopamine**, which strengthens the connection between the behavior and positive feelings. For example, after completing a morning walk, take a moment to reflect on how good you feel, or give yourself a mental pat on the back. This practice helps build positive associations with the behavior.

13.2 The Psychology of Behavior Change

13.2.1 The Stages of Change Model

The **Stages of Change Model** (also known as the **Transtheoretical Model**) is a framework that describes the process individuals go through when changing a behavior. Understanding these stages can help you identify where you are in your journey and determine the best strategies to move forward.

- **Precontemplation**: In this stage, an individual is not yet considering a change. They may not see the need to change or may be unaware of the negative consequences of their current behavior. For example, someone might not yet recognize the impact of a sedentary lifestyle on their health.

- **Contemplation**: In the **contemplation** stage, the individual is aware of the need for change and is considering making a change but has not yet taken action. They may feel ambivalent, weighing the pros and cons of changing their behavior. For instance, they may want to start exercising but feel uncertain about finding the time.

- **Preparation**: During the **preparation** stage, the individual is planning to take action soon—typically within the next **month**. They may begin to make small changes, such as researching exercise options or buying a pair of running shoes. This stage involves setting goals and developing a plan for change.

- **Action**: In the **action** stage, the individual actively implements the behavior change. For example, they might start going for daily walks, tracking their food intake, or joining a fitness class. This stage requires **effort**, **commitment**, and **support** to maintain motivation.

- **Maintenance**: The **maintenance** stage involves sustaining the new behavior over time, typically for **six months or more**. During this stage, the behavior has become part of the individual's routine, but they must remain vigilant to avoid relapsing into old habits. Building a support system, developing resilience, and continuing to focus on the benefits of the behavior are crucial in this stage.

- **Relapse**: **Relapse** is a common part of the behavior change process, where the individual returns to their old behavior. It's important to view relapse not as a failure but as a learning opportunity. Identifying the triggers that led to relapse and developing strategies to handle them in the future helps individuals continue progressing toward their goals.

13.2.2 The Role of Motivation in Habit Building

Motivation is often the driving force that initiates behavior change, but it's not always consistent or reliable. Understanding the different types of motivation and how to harness them can help you sustain positive behaviors long-term.

- **Intrinsic vs. Extrinsic Motivation: Intrinsic motivation** comes from within and is driven by personal satisfaction, enjoyment, or a sense of accomplishment. For example, exercising because you enjoy the way it makes you feel is intrinsic motivation. **Extrinsic motivation** is driven by external factors, such as rewards, recognition, or avoiding negative outcomes. For example, exercising to lose weight or impress others is extrinsic motivation. Intrinsic motivation is more effective for sustaining habits over time because it is inherently linked to personal values and enjoyment.

- **Finding Your "Why"**: To create lasting behavior change, it's important to identify your deeper **"why"**— the reason you want to develop a particular habit. For example, your "why" for eating healthier might be to have more energy to play with your children or to reduce your risk of illness. Connecting your habits to a meaningful purpose helps you stay motivated, even when it's challenging.

- **The Role of Discipline**: While motivation can fluctuate, **discipline** is what helps you maintain habits when motivation wanes. Discipline involves committing to your goals and taking action, even when you don't feel motivated. By focusing on the routine and creating a structure that supports your goals—such as scheduling workouts at a consistent time or meal prepping each week—you can ensure that healthy behaviors continue even during periods of low motivation.

13.3 Building Lasting Habits: Strategies and Techniques

13.3.1 Habit Stacking and Anchoring

Habit stacking and **anchoring** are powerful techniques for building new habits by connecting them to existing routines. These methods help create a sequence of behaviors that makes it easier to incorporate new habits into your daily life.

- **How Habit Stacking Works: Habit stacking** involves identifying a habit you already do regularly and using it as a cue for a new habit. For example, if you want to build a habit of drinking more water, stack it onto your morning coffee routine: "After I make my morning coffee, I will drink a glass of water." By linking the new habit to an established routine, you create a reliable trigger that helps you remember and practice the new behavior.

- **Anchoring to Positive Experiences: Anchoring** a new habit to a positive experience helps create a positive association with the behavior. For example, if you want to start meditating, you could anchor the habit to a relaxing part of your day, such as right after a warm shower. Associating the new habit with a positive experience helps increase motivation and enjoyment, making it more likely that the habit will stick.

13.3.2 Implementation Intentions

Implementation intentions are specific "if-then" plans that help you act on your intentions, especially when facing obstacles. By having a plan in place for how you will respond to challenges, you are more likely to follow through with your goals.

- **Creating If-Then Plans**: An **implementation intention** involves identifying a potential barrier and creating a plan for how you will overcome it. For example, if you want to exercise regularly but often feel too tired after work, create an implementation intention: "If I feel too tired after work, then I will do a 10-minute yoga session instead of skipping exercise entirely." This approach helps you stay consistent, even when obstacles arise.

- **Overcoming Temptations**: Implementation intentions are also useful for managing **temptations**. For example, if you're trying to reduce sugar intake, create a plan for handling cravings: "If I crave something sweet, then I will eat a piece of fruit instead of candy." Having a predetermined response to temptations makes it easier to stay on track.

13.3.3 Designing an Environment That Supports Habits

Your **environment** can either support or hinder habit formation. Designing your environment to make healthy choices more accessible and convenient is a powerful strategy for building sustainable habits.

- **Reducing Friction for Healthy Habits: Reducing friction** means making it easier to engage in the desired behavior. For example, if you want to work out in the morning, lay out your exercise clothes the night before. If you want to eat healthier, prepare nutritious meals in advance and keep healthy snacks visible and easily accessible. By reducing the effort required to engage in healthy behaviors, you increase the likelihood of following through.

- **Increasing Friction for Unhealthy Habits**: Conversely, increasing friction for unhealthy habits makes them less appealing. For example, if you're trying to cut back on late-night snacking, keep tempting foods out of sight or place them in a hard-to-reach location. Making it more inconvenient to engage in unhealthy behaviors helps reduce their frequency.

- **Visual Cues and Reminders: Visual cues** are powerful triggers for habit formation. Use visual reminders to reinforce your health goals, such as placing a **water bottle** on your desk, a **motivational quote** on your mirror, or a **fruit bowl** on the kitchen counter. Visual cues serve as constant reminders of your intentions and help prompt the desired behavior.

13.4 Overcoming Common Obstacles to Habit Formation

13.4.1 The Role of Willpower and How to Conserve It

Willpower is often described as the ability to resist temptations and make decisions that align with long-term goals. However, willpower is a limited resource, and relying solely on it to build habits can lead to burnout and failure. Understanding how to conserve willpower and use it effectively is key to sustaining positive behavior change.

- **Decision Fatigue: Decision fatigue** occurs when the mental energy required to make decisions becomes depleted throughout the day, leading to poorer choices as the day progresses. To conserve willpower, reduce the number of decisions you need to make about your habits. For example, plan meals in advance, create a workout schedule, and establish a consistent daily routine. By reducing decision-making, you free up mental energy for other important tasks.

- **Creating Automatic Routines**: The more automatic a behavior becomes, the less willpower it requires. By repeating a behavior consistently in the same context, it becomes ingrained as a habit, reducing the need for conscious effort. For example, if you make it a habit to go for a walk every evening after dinner, it eventually becomes an automatic part of your routine, requiring little to no willpower.

- **Avoiding Tempting Situations**: One way to conserve willpower is to **avoid situations** that test your self-control. For example, if you're trying to reduce your intake of sugary treats, avoid walking down the candy aisle at the grocery store. By minimizing exposure to temptations, you reduce the need to use willpower to resist them.

13.4.2 Dealing with Setbacks and Plateaus

Setbacks and **plateaus** are normal parts of the habit-building process, and how you respond to them can determine your long-term success. Learning to navigate setbacks with resilience and a growth mindset helps you stay on track.

- **Viewing Setbacks as Learning Opportunities**: Setbacks are not failures—they are opportunities to learn and grow. When you experience a setback, take time to reflect on what led to it and how you can adjust your approach moving forward. Ask yourself questions like, "What triggered this setback?" and "What can I do differently next time?" By approaching setbacks with curiosity rather than self-criticism, you can identify strategies for overcoming similar challenges in the future.

- **Adjusting Your Approach During Plateaus**: **Plateaus** occur when progress stalls, and they can be discouraging. During a plateau, it's important to evaluate your current habits and determine whether adjustments are needed. For example, if you've stopped seeing progress with your exercise routine, consider changing the type of exercise, increasing intensity, or trying a new activity to challenge your body in different ways. Plateaus are a natural part of the process, and adjusting your approach helps you continue progressing.

- **Maintaining Self-Compassion**: Practicing **self-compassion** is crucial when dealing with setbacks and plateaus. It's easy to become frustrated or discouraged, but self-criticism often leads to giving up. Instead, treat yourself with kindness and understanding, recognizing that behavior change is a journey that involves ups and downs. Remind yourself that setbacks are part of the process and that you are capable of overcoming them.

13.5 Creating a Lifestyle That Supports Long-Term Health

13.5.1 Integrating Habits into Your Identity

For habits to be truly sustainable, they must become part of your **identity**—the way you see yourself. When a habit aligns with your self-identity, it becomes a natural and enduring part of your lifestyle.

- **Identity-Based Habits**: Instead of focusing solely on what you want to achieve, focus on who you want to become. For example, instead of setting a goal to "exercise three times a week," identify yourself as "an active person" who prioritizes movement. This shift in focus makes it easier to maintain the behavior because it aligns with your identity. When you see yourself as a healthy person, making healthy choices becomes part of who you are.

- **Affirmations to Reinforce Identity: Affirmations** are positive statements that help reinforce your desired identity. Use affirmations to remind yourself of the type of person you are becoming. For example, "I am someone who takes care of my body," or "I am consistent in making choices that support my health." Repeating these affirmations helps strengthen your self-identity and supports the formation of lasting habits.

- **Celebrating Who You Are Becoming**: Take time to celebrate the person you are becoming, not just the milestones you achieve. Recognize the positive changes in your behaviors, attitudes, and mindset, and take pride in the progress you are making. Celebrating your growth helps reinforce your new identity and motivates you to continue on your path.

13.5.2 Balancing Flexibility and Consistency

Building a sustainable lifestyle requires a balance between **consistency** and **flexibility**. While consistency is key to habit formation, flexibility ensures that your lifestyle remains adaptable and enjoyable.

- **The Importance of Routine**: Having a **routine** helps create consistency, making it easier to repeat desired behaviors until they become habits. A consistent routine provides structure, reduces decision-making, and makes it more likely that you will follow through with your intentions. For example, having a set time each day for **exercise**, **meal preparation**, or **self-care** helps ensure that these activities become a regular part of your life.

- **Allowing for Flexibility**: Life is unpredictable, and being too rigid with your routine can lead to burnout or frustration when unexpected events occur. Allowing for flexibility means understanding that it's okay to adjust your habits when needed. For example, if you miss a workout because of a busy day, find a different time to move, or do a shorter session. Flexibility allows you to adapt your habits to fit different situations, ensuring that they remain sustainable over time.

- **The 80/20 Rule**: The **80/20 rule** is a helpful approach to balancing consistency and flexibility. This rule suggests that you focus on making healthy choices **80%** of the time, while allowing for **20%** flexibility for indulgences or less structured moments. This approach helps you maintain balance without feeling restricted, making it easier to stick to your habits long-term.

13.5.3 Creating a Support System for Sustainability

A **support system** is an essential component of building and maintaining sustainable habits. Having people around you who encourage and support your health goals makes it easier to stay on track and motivated.

- **Accountability Partners**: An **accountability partner** is someone who shares your health goals and is committed to helping you stay on track. Whether it's a friend, family member, or coworker, having someone to check in with regularly provides motivation and accountability. You can share your progress, celebrate successes, and work through challenges together.

- **Joining Health Communities**: Being part of a **health community** provides a sense of belonging and support. Whether it's a **fitness class**, an **online wellness group**, or a **local support group**, being surrounded by like-minded individuals helps reinforce your commitment to your health goals. Communities provide encouragement, shared experiences, and a space to learn from others.

- **Seeking Professional Guidance**: Working with a **health coach, dietitian**, or **therapist** can provide valuable guidance and support for building sustainable habits. Professionals can help you develop personalized strategies, navigate obstacles, and provide accountability as you work toward your goals. Seeking professional support ensures that you have the tools and resources needed for long-term success.

Chapter 14: Mastering Nutrition for Sustainable Weight Loss and Health

14.1 Understanding Nutrition Fundamentals

14.1.1 What is Nutrition and Why Is It Important?

Nutrition is the process of providing or obtaining the food necessary for health and growth. It plays a vital role in maintaining overall health, energy levels, and supporting bodily functions. Understanding nutrition is key to making informed food choices that promote sustainable weight loss and well-being.

- **The Role of Nutrition in Health**: Nutrition provides the **macronutrients** (carbohydrates, proteins, fats) and **micronutrients** (vitamins and minerals) that are essential for bodily functions, including energy production, tissue repair, immune function, and mental health. A balanced diet is essential for maintaining a healthy weight, reducing the risk of chronic diseases, and improving quality of life.

- **Energy Balance and Weight Management**: Weight management is largely influenced by **energy balance**, which is the relationship between the number of calories consumed and the number of calories expended. To lose weight, it's important to create a **caloric deficit**—consuming fewer calories than you burn. However, the quality of the calories you consume also matters, as nutrient-dense foods support metabolism, energy levels, and overall health.

14.1.2 Macronutrients: Carbohydrates, Proteins, and Fats

Macronutrients are nutrients that provide calories or energy and are needed in larger quantities. Each macronutrient plays a unique role in the body, and understanding their functions helps create a balanced diet that supports health and weight management.

- **Carbohydrates: Carbohydrates** are the body's primary source of energy. They are broken down into **glucose**, which is used by the body's cells for fuel. Carbohydrates are categorized into **simple** and **complex** carbohydrates:

  - **Simple Carbohydrates**: These are sugars found in foods like **fruits, honey,** and **table sugar**. They provide quick energy but can lead to blood sugar spikes if consumed in excess.

  - **Complex Carbohydrates**: Found in foods like **whole grains, vegetables,** and **legumes,** complex carbohydrates contain **fiber**, which aids digestion, promotes satiety, and helps stabilize blood sugar levels. Including more complex carbohydrates in the diet is beneficial for long-term health and weight management.

- **Proteins: Proteins** are essential for building and repairing tissues, making enzymes and hormones, and supporting immune function. **Amino acids** are the building blocks of protein, and they are divided into **essential** and **non-essential** amino acids. Essential amino acids must be obtained through diet, as the body cannot produce them. **High-protein foods**, such as **lean meats, poultry, fish, eggs, dairy, beans**, and **nuts**, help support muscle mass, promote satiety, and contribute to the feeling of fullness.

- **Fats: Fats** are an important macronutrient that provides energy, supports cell structure, and aids in the absorption of **fat-soluble vitamins** (A, D, E, and K). Fats are categorized into **saturated, unsaturated,** and **trans fats:**

  o **Saturated Fats:** Found in animal products like **butter** and **red meat**, these fats should be consumed in moderation to maintain cardiovascular health.

  o **Unsaturated Fats: Monounsaturated** and **polyunsaturated fats,** found in **olive oil, nuts, seeds,** and **fatty fish**, are heart-healthy and can help reduce inflammation.

  o **Trans Fats:** These are artificially created fats found in some processed foods and should be avoided, as they are associated with an increased risk of heart disease.

14.1.3 Micronutrients: Vitamins and Minerals

Micronutrients are vitamins and minerals that are required in smaller amounts but are crucial for maintaining good health and preventing deficiencies.

- **Vitamins: Vitamins** are organic compounds that support various physiological functions. They are divided into **fat-soluble** (A, D, E, K) and **water-soluble** (B-complex and C) vitamins. Each vitamin plays a specific role in health:

    - **Vitamin A:** Supports **vision, immune function,** and **skin health.**

    - **Vitamin C:** Acts as an **antioxidant,** supports **immune health,** and aids in **collagen production.**

    - **B Vitamins:** Play a key role in **energy metabolism, brain function,** and **red blood cell formation.**

    - **Vitamin D:** Helps with **calcium absorption** and supports **bone health.** It can be obtained through **sunlight exposure** as well as dietary sources like **fish** and **fortified dairy.**

- **Minerals: Minerals** such as **calcium, iron, potassium, magnesium,** and **zinc** are essential for various bodily functions, including **bone health, oxygen transport, muscle function,** and **immune**

response. Minerals are found in a wide range of foods, including **leafy greens, nuts, seeds, dairy, and whole grains.**

- **Preventing Deficiencies**: Deficiencies in vitamins and minerals can lead to various health issues. For example, **iron deficiency** can cause **anemia**, leading to **fatigue** and **weakness**. Consuming a varied diet that includes a wide range of nutrient-dense foods helps prevent deficiencies and supports overall health.

14.2 Designing a Balanced and Flexible Diet

14.2.1 The Importance of Balanced Nutrition

A **balanced diet** provides all the nutrients the body needs in appropriate proportions to maintain health, energy levels, and support bodily functions. Understanding how to design a balanced diet helps ensure that you meet your nutritional needs while also creating a sustainable approach to weight management.

- **The Plate Method**: One of the simplest ways to create balanced meals is to use the **plate method**:

  - **Half of the Plate**: Fill half of your plate with **vegetables** and **fruits**. These foods are rich in vitamins, minerals, and fiber, which help support digestion and promote satiety.

o **Quarter of the Plate:** Allocate a quarter of the plate to **lean proteins** such as **chicken, fish, tofu,** or **beans.**

o **Quarter of the Plate:** Use the remaining quarter for **complex carbohydrates** such as **whole grains** (brown rice, quinoa) or **starchy vegetables** (sweet potatoes, corn).

o **Healthy Fats:** Add a small amount of **healthy fats** from sources like **olive oil, avocado,** or **nuts.**

- **Portion Control: Portion control** is key to creating a balanced diet, especially for weight management. Consuming portions that match your energy needs helps you maintain a caloric deficit or balance, depending on your goals. Using smaller plates, being mindful of serving sizes, and listening to your body's hunger and fullness cues are effective strategies for managing portions.

- **Variety for Nutrient Diversity:** Including a wide variety of foods in your diet helps ensure that you get a broad spectrum of nutrients. Different foods contain different vitamins, minerals, and antioxidants, so a varied diet helps support overall health. Aim to include a rainbow of fruits and vegetables, diverse protein sources, and a mix of healthy fats.

14.2.2 Flexible Dieting and the 80/20 Approach

Flexible dieting is an approach that allows for **moderation** and **balance** without the need for strict restrictions. It involves creating a healthy diet that includes mostly nutrient-dense foods while also allowing for occasional indulgences, making it easier to maintain over the long term.

- **The 80/20 Rule**: The **80/20 rule** is a helpful framework for flexible dieting. This rule suggests that **80%** of your diet should consist of nutrient-dense, whole foods such as **vegetables, fruits, lean proteins**, and **whole grains**, while **20%** can include less nutrient-dense foods that you enjoy, such as **desserts, snacks**, or **alcohol**. This approach allows for balance and flexibility, helping you avoid feelings of deprivation.

- **Mindful Indulgence**: Flexible dieting encourages **mindful indulgence** rather than restriction. This means allowing yourself to enjoy your favorite foods in moderation, without guilt. For example, if you enjoy chocolate, include a small piece as part of your daily diet rather than restricting it entirely. Mindful indulgence helps reduce cravings, prevents binge eating, and makes it easier to maintain a healthy lifestyle over time.

- **Tracking Macros vs. Intuitive Eating**: Some individuals prefer to **track macronutrients** (carbs, proteins, fats) to ensure they are meeting their nutritional needs, while others prefer an **intuitive eating** approach, which involves listening to the body's hunger and fullness cues. Both approaches can be effective for different people, depending on their preferences and relationship with food. The key is to find a method that feels sustainable and aligns with your health goals.

14.3 Meal Planning, Preparation, and Cooking Skills

14.3.1 The Benefits of Meal Planning

Meal planning is an effective strategy for maintaining a balanced diet, reducing food waste, and making healthier choices throughout the week. Planning your meals in advance helps ensure that you have **nutritious options** available, reduces the temptation to order **takeout**, and saves time and money.

- **Weekly Meal Planning**: Set aside time each week to plan your meals. Start by deciding what you want to eat for **breakfast, lunch, dinner**, and **snacks**. Consider your schedule and choose meals that are practical for each day—quick options for busy days and more elaborate recipes when you have more time. Write down a **shopping list** based on your meal plan to ensure you have all the ingredients you need.

- **Batch Cooking and Meal Prep: Batch cooking** involves preparing larger quantities of food that can be used throughout the week. For example, cook a large pot of **soup, chili**, or **stew** that can be portioned out for multiple meals. **Meal prep** also involves preparing ingredients in advance—such as **chopping vegetables, cooking grains**, or **marinating proteins**—so that meals can be assembled quickly during the week. This reduces cooking time and ensures that healthy meals are always available.

- **Building Balanced Meals**: When planning meals, aim to include a **balance of macronutrients**—carbohydrates, proteins, and fats—along with plenty of vegetables. This ensures that your meals are filling, nutritious, and support your energy needs. For example, a balanced lunch might include **grilled chicken** (protein), **quinoa** (complex carbohydrates), **spinach and bell peppers** (vegetables), and **avocado** (healthy fats).

14.3.2 Cooking Skills for Healthy Eating

Cooking at home is one of the best ways to take control of your nutrition. Developing basic **cooking skills** allows you to prepare healthy, delicious meals and make informed choices about ingredients.

- **Learning Basic Cooking Techniques**: Start by learning basic cooking techniques, such as **baking, grilling, steaming**, and **sautéing**. These methods are generally healthier than **frying**, as they require less added fat and help preserve the nutrients in your food. Experiment with different cooking techniques to find what you enjoy and to add variety to your meals.

- **Using Herbs and Spices: Herbs and spices** are a great way to add flavor to your meals without extra calories, sugar, or salt. Experiment with different herbs (e.g., **basil, rosemary, cilantro**) and spices (e.g., **cumin, paprika, turmeric**) to create a variety of flavors and make your meals more enjoyable. Using herbs and spices also adds health benefits, as many have **anti-inflammatory** and **antioxidant** properties.

- **Healthy Cooking Substitutions**: Making small substitutions can significantly improve the nutritional value of your meals. For example, replace **sour cream** with **Greek yogurt**, use **applesauce** instead of **butter** in baking, or swap **white rice** for **quinoa** or **brown rice**. These substitutions help reduce calories, increase fiber, and improve the overall nutrient profile of your meals.

14.3.3 Reading and Understanding Food Labels

Food labels provide important information about the nutritional content of packaged foods, helping you make informed choices about what to include in your diet.

- **Key Components of a Food Label**: Understanding the key components of a food label can help you assess the quality of a product:

  - **Serving Size**: The serving size listed on the label is the amount that all the nutritional information refers to. Be mindful of serving sizes, as many packaged foods contain multiple servings.

  - **Calories**: **Calories** are a measure of energy, and understanding how many calories are in a serving helps you determine whether the food fits into your daily energy needs.

  - **Macronutrient Breakdown**: Look at the amounts of **carbohydrates, proteins**, and

fats per serving. Be mindful of added **sugars** and try to choose products with minimal added sugar. Pay attention to the types of fats listed—**unsaturated fats** are generally healthier, while **trans fats** should be avoided.

- Ingredient List: The **ingredient list** provides insight into the quality of the product. Ingredients are listed in descending order by weight, so the first few ingredients make up the bulk of the product. Look for **whole, recognizable ingredients**, and avoid products with **long lists of artificial additives**.

- **Identifying Hidden Sugars**: Sugar is often added to processed foods, sometimes under different names. Look for **hidden sugars** such as **high-fructose corn syrup, sucrose, maltose**, or **honey** on the ingredient list. Choosing products with little to no added sugar helps support stable energy levels and weight management.

14.4 The Role of Mindful Eating in Nutrition

14.4.1 What is Mindful Eating?

Mindful eating is the practice of paying attention to the experience of eating, including the taste, texture, and aroma of food, as well as your body's hunger and fullness cues. It involves being present during meals, eating without distractions, and developing a positive relationship with food.

- **The Benefits of Mindful Eating: Mindful eating** helps improve your awareness of what, why, and how much you're eating, leading to better food choices and portion control. It also helps you appreciate and savor your food, which can enhance satisfaction and reduce the likelihood of overeating. By paying attention to your body's hunger and fullness signals, you learn to eat when you're hungry and stop when you're satisfied, rather than eating out of habit or emotion.

- **Practicing Mindfulness During Meals**: To practice mindful eating, start by eliminating distractions—turn off the TV, put away your phone, and focus solely on your meal. Take small bites, chew slowly, and notice the flavors, textures, and aromas of the food. Pay attention to how your body feels as you eat, and stop eating when you feel comfortably full, rather than stuffed. Mindful eating helps you enjoy your meals more fully and develop a healthier relationship with food.

14.4.2 Emotional Eating vs. Physical Hunger

Emotional eating is eating in response to emotions—such as stress, boredom, or sadness—rather than physical hunger. Understanding the difference between **emotional** and

physical hunger helps you make more mindful food choices and manage cravings in a healthy way.

- **Identifying Physical Hunger: Physical hunger** is characterized by physical sensations, such as a growling stomach, a feeling of emptiness, or low energy. It comes on gradually and can be satisfied with a variety of foods. When you're physically hungry, you are likely to feel satisfied after eating.

- **Recognizing Emotional Hunger: Emotional hunger**, on the other hand, is often sudden and specific. You may crave a particular type of food, such as **sweets** or **junk food**, and the urge to eat may feel urgent. Emotional hunger is usually not satisfied by eating, and it often leads to feelings of guilt or regret afterward. Recognizing emotional hunger helps you pause and consider whether you're truly hungry or if you're using food to cope with emotions.

- **Coping with Emotional Triggers**: Instead of turning to food to cope with emotions, develop alternative **coping strategies**. For example, if you're feeling stressed, try **deep breathing, journaling, taking a walk**, or **talking to a friend**. Creating a list of activities that help you feel calm or uplifted can provide healthier ways to cope with emotional triggers without relying on food.

14.4.3 Listening to Hunger and Fullness Cues

Learning to listen to your body's **hunger** and **fullness cues** is an important aspect of both mindful eating and sustainable weight management. It helps you eat in response to your body's needs rather than external cues, such as the time of day or portion sizes.

- **The Hunger Scale**: The **hunger scale** is a tool that helps you gauge your level of hunger and fullness. Imagine a scale from **1 to 10**, where **1** represents extreme hunger, **5** is neutral, and **10** is extreme fullness. Aim to eat when you're around a **3 or 4** (feeling hungry but not starving) and stop when you're at a **6 or 7** (feeling comfortably satisfied). This helps prevent overeating and ensures that you're eating in response to true hunger.

- **Checking In During Meals**: Throughout your meal, check in with yourself to assess how you're feeling. Ask yourself if you're still hungry or if you're beginning to feel satisfied. Eating slowly and taking breaks during your meal allows your body to register fullness, helping you stop before overeating.

14.5 Managing Cravings and Emotional Eating

14.5.1 Understanding and Managing Food Cravings

Food cravings are intense desires for specific foods, often those that are high in **sugar**, **fat**, or **salt**. While cravings are a natural part of eating, understanding the root causes of cravings can help you manage them in a balanced way.

- **Common Triggers for Cravings**: **Cravings** can be triggered by a variety of factors, including:

  - **Emotions**: Stress, boredom, or sadness can trigger cravings for comfort foods.

  - **Nutrient Deficiencies**: A lack of certain nutrients (e.g., magnesium, iron) can lead to specific cravings.

  - **Environmental Cues**: Seeing or smelling certain foods can trigger cravings, even if you're not hungry.

  - **Habit**: Cravings can also be a result of habitual eating patterns, such as always having dessert after dinner.

- **Balanced Approaches to Managing Cravings**: Instead of resisting cravings entirely, it's often more effective to address them in a balanced way:

  - **Satisfy Cravings in Moderation**: Allow yourself to enjoy the food you're craving in moderation. For example, have a small piece of chocolate rather than avoiding it completely. Satisfying cravings in a mindful way can prevent overindulgence later.

  - **Identify and Address Triggers**: If you notice certain situations or emotions consistently trigger cravings, develop strategies to address those triggers. For example, if stress triggers cravings for sweets, find alternative stress-relief activities, such as **yoga** or **listening to music**.

o   **Choose Healthier Alternatives**: If you're craving something sweet, choose healthier options like **fruit, Greek yogurt**, or a small amount of **dark chocolate**. For salty cravings, opt for **air-popped popcorn or roasted nuts**. Healthier alternatives provide satisfaction without compromising your nutrition goals.

14.5.2 Emotional Eating: Breaking the Cycle

Emotional eating can lead to overeating and weight gain if not managed effectively. Breaking the cycle of emotional eating involves recognizing the triggers, finding healthier coping mechanisms, and developing a more positive relationship with food.

- **Recognizing Patterns**: Start by recognizing the patterns of emotional eating in your life. Keep a **journal** to track when you eat, what you eat, and how you're feeling at the time. This helps identify emotional triggers and develop awareness of when you're eating in response to emotions rather than hunger.

- **Developing Alternative Coping Strategies**: Instead of turning to food to cope with emotions, create a list of **alternative activities** that bring comfort or distraction. This might include **going for a walk, calling a friend, practicing meditation**, or engaging in a **hobby**. Having a list of go-to activities makes it easier to resist the urge to eat for emotional reasons.

- **Building Emotional Awareness**: Building **emotional awareness** helps you respond to your emotions in healthier ways. Practice naming your emotions when they arise and acknowledging them without judgment. For example, if you're feeling stressed, simply say to yourself, "I'm feeling stressed right now." Acknowledging your emotions allows you to address them in healthier ways without turning to food.

14.6 Creating a Sustainable Nutrition Plan for Life

14.6.1 Setting Realistic and Personalized Nutrition Goals

Creating a **sustainable nutrition plan** starts with setting realistic, achievable goals that fit your lifestyle and preferences. Personalized goals are more motivating and easier to maintain over the long term.

- **Setting SMART Goals**: Use the **SMART** criteria to set nutrition goals that are:

  o **Specific**: Clearly define what you want to achieve. For example, "I want to eat **five servings** of vegetables daily."

  o **Measurable**: Make sure your goal is measurable so you can track your progress. For example, "I will drink **eight glasses of water** each day."

  o **Achievable**: Set goals that are realistic and within your capabilities. For example, "I will cook dinner at home **four nights a week**."

  o **Relevant**: Ensure that your goals are aligned with your overall health objectives. For example, "I want to reduce my sugar intake to improve my energy levels."

- o **Time-Bound**: Set a timeframe for achieving your goal. For example, "I will achieve this goal over the next **two months**."

- **Adapting Goals Over Time**: Nutrition needs and goals may change over time, depending on factors such as **age, activity level**, or **health conditions**. Be open to adjusting your goals as needed and remain flexible. For example, if you begin a new exercise program, you may need to increase your calorie intake to support your activity.

14.6.2 Making Nutrition Enjoyable and Sustainable

To create a nutrition plan that is sustainable, it's important to find enjoyment in the foods you eat and avoid a restrictive mindset. A positive and enjoyable approach to nutrition makes it easier to maintain healthy habits for life.

- **Finding Foods You Enjoy**: Healthy eating doesn't mean eating foods you dislike. Experiment with different ingredients, flavors, and cooking methods to find **nutritious foods** that you genuinely enjoy. Including a variety of foods helps prevent boredom and makes it more likely that you will stick to your nutrition plan.

- **Avoiding Restriction and Deprivation**: Restrictive diets that eliminate entire food groups or require severe calorie reduction are difficult to maintain and can lead to **binge eating** or **unhealthy relationships** with food. Instead of restriction, focus on adding **nutrient-dense** foods to your diet while allowing for **moderate indulgence** in foods you enjoy. This balanced approach helps prevent feelings of deprivation and makes it easier to sustain healthy eating habits.

- **Creating Positive Associations with Healthy Foods**: Create positive associations with healthy foods by focusing on their benefits and how they make you feel. For example, after eating a **balanced meal**, take note of how it makes you feel energized and satisfied. Focusing on the positive outcomes of healthy eating reinforces the habit and makes it more enjoyable.

14.6.3 Nutrition as a Lifelong Practice

Nutrition is not about short-term diets or quick fixes; it's a lifelong practice that supports overall health, well-being, and quality of life. Embracing nutrition as a long-term commitment helps create a sustainable approach that evolves with you.

- **Adopting a Long-Term Perspective**: Rather than focusing on **short-term weight loss** goals, adopt a long-term perspective that prioritizes health and well-being. This means making consistent choices that support your health, even if progress seems slow at times. Remember that health is a journey, and every small positive change contributes to your long-term well-being.

- **Building a Positive Relationship with Food**: Developing a **positive relationship** with food is key to sustainable nutrition. View food as fuel that nourishes your body and supports your goals, rather than something to be feared or restricted. Practice self-compassion when you make choices that don't align perfectly with your goals, and remember that balance is the key to sustainability.

- **Evolving Your Nutrition Habits**: As you go through different stages of life, your nutrition needs and preferences may change. Be open to evolving your nutrition habits to fit your current lifestyle, health needs, and personal goals. Whether it's incorporating more **plant-based meals**, adjusting **calorie intake**, or focusing on **specific nutrients** for a health condition, remain flexible and adaptive in your approach.

Appendix: Tools and Resources for Sustainable Weight Loss and Health

A.1 Nutrition and Meal Planning Tools

A.1.1 Grocery Shopping Checklist

A well-organized grocery list helps ensure that you have everything you need for healthy meals throughout the week. Below is a sample **grocery shopping checklist** with key items that support a balanced diet:

- **Vegetables:**

- Leafy greens (spinach, kale, lettuce)
    - Broccoli, cauliflower
    - Bell peppers, carrots
    - Tomatoes, cucumbers
    - Zucchini, eggplant
- **Fruits:**
    - Apples, bananas, berries
    - Oranges, grapefruit, pineapple
    - Grapes, mango, pears
- **Proteins:**
    - Chicken breast, lean beef, fish
    - Tofu, tempeh
    - Eggs
    - Beans, lentils, chickpeas
    - Nuts, seeds (almonds, chia, sunflower)
- **Grains and Starches:**
    - Brown rice, quinoa, bulgur
    - Whole wheat bread, wraps
    - Oats
    - Sweet potatoes, potatoes
- **Dairy or Alternatives:**
    - Greek yogurt, cottage cheese

o   Milk (dairy, almond, soy)

o   Cheese

- **Healthy Fats**:

o   Olive oil, avocado oil

o   Avocados

o   Nut butter (peanut, almond)

- **Herbs and Spices**:

o   Fresh or dried herbs (basil, cilantro, parsley)

o   Spices (cumin, paprika, turmeric, cinnamon)

- **Snacks**:

o   Fresh fruit, cut vegetables

o   Hummus

o   Dark chocolate (70% or higher)

- **Pantry Staples**:

o   Canned beans, tomatoes

o   Whole grain pasta

o   Broth or stock

Use this checklist to customize your weekly shopping based on your meal plan.

A.1.2 Meal Planning Template

Use the following template to plan your weekly meals. This helps ensure balanced nutrition and saves time:

Day	Breakfast	Lunch	Dinner	Snacks
Monday	Overnight oats with berries	Grilled chicken salad	Stir-fried vegetables with tofu	Greek yogurt with honey
Tuesday	Scrambled eggs with spinach	Turkey wrap with veggies	Baked salmon with quinoa	Apple slices with almond butter
Wednesday	Smoothie (banana, spinach, protein)	Lentil soup	Chicken fajitas	Carrot sticks with hummus
Thursday	Greek yogurt with granola	Quinoa bowl with chickpeas	Grilled shrimp and veggies	Fresh berries
Friday	Whole grain toast with avocado	Leftover stir-fry	Spaghetti with marinara sauce and turkey meatballs	Cottage cheese with pineapple
Saturday	Omelet with bell peppers	Veggie wrap	Veggie curry with brown rice	Mixed nuts
Sunday	Protein pancakes	Mixed greens	Homemade pizza with veggies	Dark chocolate square

Day	Breakfast	Lunch	Dinner	Snacks
		with salmon		

A.1.3 Recipe Modification Tips

For those interested in modifying traditional recipes to be healthier, here are some helpful substitutions:

- **Replace white flour** with **whole wheat flour** or **oat flour** for added fiber.

- **Use Greek yogurt** instead of **sour cream** to reduce calories and fat.

- **Bake** or **grill** instead of frying to reduce oil and calorie intake.

- **Use applesauce** or **mashed bananas** as a substitute for butter in baked goods for moisture and sweetness.

A.2 Fitness and Physical Activity Tools

A.2.1 Workout Planner Template

This **workout planner** template helps keep your physical activity routine structured and consistent. Customize it based on your fitness goals and preferences.

Day	Activity Type	Duration	Notes/Comments
Monday	Cardio (Running)	30 minutes	Focus on intervals

Day	Activity Type	Duration	Notes/Comments
Tuesday	Strength Training (Upper Body)	45 minutes	Free weights at the gym
Wednesday	Yoga	20 minutes	Relaxation and flexibility
Thursday	Cardio (Cycling)	40 minutes	Outdoor route, moderate pace
Friday	Strength Training (Lower Body)	45 minutes	Use resistance bands
Saturday	Hiking	60 minutes	With friends
Sunday	Rest/Light Stretching	-	Self-care, gentle stretches

A.2.2 Tracking Physical Progress

Tracking your progress helps stay motivated. Use the following metrics:

- **Workout consistency**: How many days a week you exercised.

- **Increased endurance**: Time it takes to run or walk a mile.

- **Strength gains**: Weight lifted, number of reps or sets completed.

- **Flexibility improvements**: Ability to reach and hold stretches.

- **Energy levels**: How you feel before and after workouts.

A.3 Mindful Eating and Emotional Health Tools

A.3.1 Hunger and Fullness Scale

This **Hunger and Fullness Scale** helps you tune into your body's cues:

Scale	Description
1	Extremely hungry, dizzy, irritable
2	Very hungry, stomach growling, low energy
3	Hungry, ready to eat
4	Slightly hungry, can eat soon
5	Neutral, neither hungry nor full
6	Satisfied, comfortable
7	Slightly full, but not uncomfortable
8	Full, could have eaten a little less
9	Very full, uncomfortable
10	Extremely full, feeling stuffed

Aim to eat when you're around a **3 or 4** and stop when you're at a **6 or 7**.

A.3.2 Emotional Eating Tracker

Tracking your emotional eating can help you recognize triggers and patterns:

Date	Emotion (e.g., stress, boredom)	Food Craved	Situation/Trigger	Alternative Strategy Used	Notes
July 5	Stress	Chocolate	Deadline at work	Went for a walk	Craving decreased
July 8	Boredom	Chips	Watching TV	Read a book instead	Managed to avoid snacking

A.4 Recommended Resources

A.4.1 Books and Reading Materials

- **"Atomic Habits" by James Clear**: A guide to building good habits and breaking bad ones.

- **"The Power of Habit" by Charles Duhigg**: Explores the science of habit formation.

- **"Mindless Eating" by Brian Wansink**: Insight into the psychology of eating and how to make better food choices.

- **"Intuitive Eating" by Evelyn Tribole and Elyse Resch**: Helps develop a positive relationship with food through mindful and intuitive eating practices.

A.4.2 Apps for Tracking Nutrition and Fitness

- **MyFitnessPal**: A comprehensive app for tracking food intake, exercise, and calories.

- **Fitbit**: Tracks steps, sleep, and physical activity, and integrates with health goals.

- **Headspace**: A meditation app that helps with stress management and mindfulness.

- **WaterMinder**: Helps track water intake to stay hydrated throughout the day.

A.4.3 Websites and Blogs

- **Nutrition.gov**: Provides credible nutrition information, recipes, and dietary guidelines.

- **EatRight.org**: The website of the Academy of Nutrition and Dietetics, offering healthy eating resources.

- **Cooking Light Blog**: Offers recipes, meal ideas, and tips for healthy cooking.

A.5 Templates for Goal Setting and Progress Tracking

A.5.1 SMART Goal Worksheet

Use this worksheet to set **SMART goals** for weight loss, health, or wellness:

Goal Element	Details
Specific	What exactly do you want to achieve?
Measurable	How will you measure your progress?

Goal Element	Details
Achievable	Is this goal realistic?
Relevant	How does this goal align with your broader health objectives?
Time-Bound	What is your deadline for achieving this goal?

Example Goal: **"I will exercise for 30 minutes, 4 times a week, for the next three months to improve my cardiovascular health and reduce stress."**

A.5.2 Habit Tracker Template

Tracking habits helps you stay consistent and see progress over time. Use the following template to track your daily habits:

Habit	Mon	Tue	Wed	Thu	Fri	Sat	Sun
Drink 8 glasses of water	✓	✓	✓	✗	✓	✓	✓
Morning stretch routine	✓	✓	✓	✓	✓	✗	✓
No sugary snacks	✓	✗	✓	✓	✗	✓	✓

A.6 Frequently Asked Questions (FAQs)

A.6.1 Common Questions on Weight Loss and Nutrition

1. **How do I calculate my daily calorie needs?**

   - You can use an online **Basal Metabolic Rate (BMR)** calculator to estimate your daily calorie needs based on your age, gender, weight, height, and activity level.

2. **Is it necessary to cut out carbs to lose weight?**

    o **No.** Carbs are an important source of energy. Instead of cutting them out, focus on consuming **complex carbohydrates** like whole grains, legumes, and vegetables, which provide fiber and nutrients.

3. **How can I deal with cravings without giving in?**

    o Practice **mindful indulgence**, drink water to assess if it's thirst, or try healthier alternatives. Identifying emotional triggers for cravings can also help you address the root cause.

4. **Do I need to exercise every day to lose weight?**

    o **Not necessarily.** Aim for **150 minutes of moderate exercise per week**. Incorporate a mix of **cardio, strength training,** and **flexibility exercises**. Rest days are important for recovery.

A.6.2 Questions on Motivation and Mindset

1. **How do I stay motivated on my weight loss journey?**

    o Set **small, achievable goals,** celebrate your progress, and remind yourself of your "why." Surround yourself with supportive people, and remember that motivation can fluctuate—**discipline** is key to consistency.

2. **What if I relapse and return to old habits?**

o   **Relapse is part of the journey**. Reflect on what led to it, learn from the experience, and recommit to your goals. Practice **self-compassion**—progress is not linear.

A.7 Glossary of Terms

A.7.1 Nutrition Terms

- **Macronutrients**: Nutrients needed in large amounts—**carbohydrates, proteins, fats**.

- **Micronutrients**: Nutrients needed in smaller amounts—**vitamins and minerals**.

- **Caloric Deficit**: Consuming fewer calories than your body needs to create energy for weight loss.

A.7.2 Fitness Terms

- **Cardiovascular Exercise**: Exercises that raise your heart rate, such as **running** or **cycling**.

- **Strength Training**: Exercises that build muscle strength, such as **weight lifting** or **bodyweight exercises**.

- **Flexibility**: The range of motion in your joints; improved by stretching or activities like **yoga**.